THE PARENT'S SURVIVAL GUIDE TO
DAYCARE INFECTIONS

Edited by
Leigh B. Grossman, MD

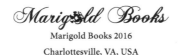

Marigold Books 2016
Charlottesville, VA, USA

ISBN: 978-0-9974999-0-2

Library of Congress Control Number: 2016915906
Marigold Books, Charlottesville, VA

Cover by Watermark Design, Charlottesville, VA
Book Development & Production by Chenille Books, Charlottesville, VA

*For my grandsons, Brock and Taylor,
who role model
what healthy daycare and
preschool years can and should be
for all children.*

CONTENTS

CONTRIBUTING AUTHORS

STUART P. ADLER, M.D.
Director, Cytomegalovirus Research Foundation, Inc.
Richmond, Virginia

SUSAN M. ANDERSON, M.D.
Associate Professor of Clinical Pediatrics
University of Virginia Health System
Charlottesville, Virginia

JAMES CHRISTOPHER DAY, M.D.
Assistant Professor of Pediatric Infectious Disease
Children's Mercy Hospital & Clinics
Kansas City, Missouri

JEFFREY R. DONOWITZ, M.D.
Fellow, Pediatric Infectious Disease
Virginia Commonwealth University Health System
Richmond, Virginia

ANNE A. GERSHON, M.D.
Professor of Pediatric Infectious Disease
Columbia University College of Physicians and Surgeons
New York, New York

CHARLES M. GINSBURG, M.D.
Marilyn R. Corrigan Distinguished Chair of Pediatric Research
Senior Associate Dean
University of Texas Southwestern Medical Center
Dallas, Texas

LEIGH B. GROSSMAN, M.D.
Medical Alumni Professor of Pediatric Infectious Disease
Associate Dean for International Programs
University of Virginia Health System
Charlottesville, Virginia

SCOTT A. HALPERIN, M.D.
Professor of Pediatrics and Microbiology and Immunology
Head, Pediatric Infectious Disease
Director, Canadian Center for Vaccinology
Dalhousie University
Halifax, Nova Scotia, Canada

MARGARET R. HAMMERSCHLAG, M.D.
Professor of Pediatrics and Medicine
Director, Pediatric Infectious Disease Training Program
SUNY Downstate Medical Center
Brooklyn, New York

GREGORY F. HAYDEN, M.D.
Professor Emeritus of Pediatrics
University of Virginia Health System
Charlottesville, Virginia

VINCENT IANNELLI, M.D.
Associate Professor of Pediatrics
Southwestern Medical School in Dallas
Rowlett, Texas

MARY ANNE JACKSON, M.D.
Director, Division of Pediatric Infectious Disease
Associate Chair of Community and Regional Pediatric Collaboration
Children's Mercy Hospital
Kansas City, Missouri

RICHARD F. JACOBS, M.D.
Robert H. Fiser Jr., M.D. Chair of Pediatric Infectious Disease
Professor and Chair of Pediatrics
Arkansas Children's Hospital
Little Rock, Arkansas

BARBARA A. JANTAUSCH, M.D.
Professor of Pediatric Infectious Disease
Children's National Health System
Washington, DC

SHELDON L. KAPLAN, M.D.
Professor and Vice-Chair of Pediatrics
Head, Section of Pediatric Infectious Disease
Baylor College of Medicine
Texas Children's Hospital
Houston, Texas

DAVID A. KAUFMAN, M.D.
Professor of Pediatric Neonatology
University of Virginia Health System
Charlottesville, Virginia

WILLIAM C. KOCH, M.D.
Associate Professor of Pediatric Infectious Disease
Virginia Commonwealth University Medical Center
Richmond, Virginia

MARIAN G. MICHAELS, M.D., M.P.H.
Professor of Pediatrics and Surgery
Division of Pediatric Infectious Diseases
Children's Hospital of Pittsburgh of UPMC
Pittsburgh, Pennsylvania

CHRISANNA M. MINK, M.D.
Professor of Pediatric Infectious Disease
Director, KIDS Clinic
Harbor-UCLA Pediatrics
Torrance, California

JONATHAN P. MOORMAN, M.D., PhD
Professor and Chief of Infectious Disease
East Tennessee State University College of Medicine
Johnson City, Tennessee

TRUDY V. MURPHY, M.D.
Team Lead, Vaccine Research and Policy
National Center for HIV/AIDS, Viral Hepatitis, STD,
  and TB Prevention (NCHHSTP)
Centers for Disease Control and Prevention
Atlanta, Georgia

MICHAEL F. REIN, M.D.
Professor Emeritus of Infectious Disease
University of Virginia Health System
Charlottesville, Virginia

KAREN S. RHEUBAN, M.D.
Professor of Pediatric Cardiology
Senior Associate Dean for Continuing Medical Education
University of Virginia Health System
Charlottesville, Virginia

WILLIAM J. RODRIGUEZ, M.D., PhD
Science Director, Office of Pediatric Therapeutics
Office of the Commissioner, Food & Drug Administration
Silver Spring, Maryland

THERESA A. SCHLAGER, M.D.
Professor of Pediatrics and Emergency Medicine
University of Virginia Health System
Charlottesville, Virginia

GWENDOLYN B. SCOTT, M.D.
Professor of Pediatrics
Director, Division of Pediatric Infectious Disease and Immunology
University of Miami Miller School of Medicine
Miami, Florida

EUGENE D. SHAPIRO, M.D.
Professor of Pediatrics, Epidemiology
  and Investigative Medicine
Associate Chair, Department of Pediatrics
Yale University School of Medicine
New Haven, Connecticut

ZIAD M. SHEHAB, M.D.
Professor of Pediatrics and Pathology
Head, Division of Pediatric Infectious Disease
The University of Arizona
Tucson, Arizona

STEPHANIE H. STOVALL, M.D.
Director, Division of Pediatric Infectious Disease
Golisano Children's Hospital of Southwest Florida
Fort Myers, Florida

CIRO V. SUMAYA, M.D., M.P.H.T.M.
Founding Dean and Professor of Health Policy and Management
School of Rural Public Health
Texas A & M Health Science Center
College Station, Texas

TANIA A. THOMAS, M.D.
Assistant Professor of Infectious Disease and International Health
Virginia Department of Health State Consultant for Pediatric TB
University of Virginia Health System
Charlottesville, Virginia

PATRICIA TREADWELL, M.D.
Professor of Pediatrics and Dermatology
Indiana University School of Medicine
Indianapolis, Indiana

RONALD B. TURNER, M.D.
Professor of Pediatric Infectious Disease
University of Virginia Health System
Charlottesville, Virginia

LINDA A. WAGGONER-FOUNTAIN, M.D., M.ED.
Associate Professor of Pediatric Infectious Disease
University of Virginia Health System
Charlottesville, Virginia

DAVID A. WHITING, M.D.
Director of The Hair and Skin Research and Treatment Center
Baylor Scott & White University Medical Center
Dallas, Texas

RICHARD J. WHITLEY, M.D.
Loeb Eminent Scholar Chair of Pediatrics, Medicine, and Microbiology
University of Alabama School of Medicine
Birmingham, Alabama

TERRY YAMAUCHI, M.D.
Inaugural Professor of Pediatrics
Clinton School of Public Services
University of Arkansas for Medical Sciences
Little Rock, Arkansas

QUICK REFERENCES

VIGNETTES

FOREWORD

Parenting is one of life's most important, enjoyable, and ful-
filling adventures. Parents provide nourishment, nurturance,
and protection for the children whose lives unfold before them.
Parents are supported in rearing their children by family, community, and services such as child health providers, daycare
centers, and home daycare providers. *The Parent's Survival
Guide to Daycare Infections* is another excellent support.

Even though infectious disease is part and parcel of all human
life, new parents can be taken off guard when their child has
the first viral or bacterial illness. Working together with their
healthcare provider, they learn how to obtain medical assessment and care. It is equally critical that they learn how their
daycare handles illness. This survival guide helps parents step
by step and gives them a clear understanding of daycare policies
and services around illness.

Parents can be baffled – even exasperated – by their child's
third, fourth, or fifth cold or stomach bug in a year. They
wonder what they or their daycare center or home daycare
provider should be doing differently to keep their child well.
This book explains to families that most children do have five
to six infections per year and that most of these are self-limited.
The book helps families to understand that when their young
child does get sick with a series of minor illnesses, it is usually
not a sign of some serious underlying condition. It is, in fact,
par for the course. The book details for parents how the human
body develops immunity through exposure to wide a variety of
infectious agents.

This wonderful book gives parents essential information about
infectious diseases and how to deal with the inevitability of
colds, stomach "bugs," rashes and even the rare, serious infectious illness. Within the book's pages, Dr. Leigh Grossman and
a talented group of experts discuss the key features of common
and uncommon infectious diseases. They teach about how
viruses and bacteria can affect different parts of a child's body
causing upper or lower respiratory problems, diarrhea or vomiting, lethargy or irritability. The experts discuss fever and other
responses that the human body uses to respond to infection.

In a detailed A to Z reference, parents can find the most authoritative information on the courses of contagious diseases that affect young children. They learn which diseases their children are most likely to encounter and which illnesses are very unusual in developed countries like the United States. They learn which diseases are preventable by vaccines. They read about treatment choices and about how long their child will need to be out of contact with other children.

Parents want to be prepared and informed and they want to be responsible members of their community. Dr. Grossman and her co-authors provide parents with excellent documentation on the role of vaccines. This book outlines key information about pertussis, tetanus, diphtheria, polio, H. influenza, meningococcus, pneumococcus, rotavirus, hepatitis, measles, mumps, rubella, and influenza. The book also explains to parents how critical it is for adults who care for children to be properly immunized. Parents who read this book are armed with all the proper information they need to counter any anti-vaccine arguments they may hear about on TV or read on the internet.

This book is packed with information about how families can be responsible members of the community when their child does contract an infectious disease. By outlining the information on recommended exclusion policies and the importance of alternative care planning, the book helps parents play their essential roles in keeping the community safe and healthy.

The book also includes excellent sections about the inclusion into daycare settings of children who have long-term illnesses, chronic infections, and disabilities. This reassuring material is helpful for all families to understand, and enriches the lives of everyone involved in the daycare experience.

Keeping our children healthy and safe is all parents' goal. Dr. Grossman and her colleagues have done a great service with this book to make sure that young children stay healthy, grow well, and achieve their best potential.

Judith S. Palfrey, MD
T. Berry Brazelton Professor of Pediatrics
Harvard Medical School
Boston, Massachusetts

PREFACE

So, after nine months of pregnancy and the delivery, you are home, thrilled to be holding your new baby, and looking forward to the time at home to be a parent. And then the daycare world begins to loom large. Or, maybe you haven't delivered yet and are trying to answer these questions ahead of time. Or, maybe the daycare waitlist time is so long that you want to sign up for your baby's place as soon as possible.

The lingering thoughts for anyone working outside the home include:

- How can I find the right daycare for my baby?
- How old should my baby be before we take her/him to a daycare center?
- What should I look for in the centers that I plan to visit?
- What can we do to minimize our baby's infections at daycare?

These and many other questions are normal, reasonable and important. You and 12 million other parents of children under the age of five in the United States use regular daycare for all or part of the week.

The term "daycare" has multiple meanings. A daycare center can be an in-home daycare usually caring for fewer than six children; a large family child care home with seven to twelve children with variable licensing requirements, or a daycare center or preschool that cares for more than 13 children and has to perform at or above the state regulated standards. Regardless of the kind of daycare or preschool setting, all children cared for outside of the home with children from other families will have a higher chance of getting an infection at daycare, have more frequent infections during the daycare and preschool years, and will likely bring home these germs and infect parents and siblings.

Most of the infections are minor viral infections and ones that all children will sooner or later be exposed to. Most of the time, child will develop a minor infectious illness and subsequently gain immunity that is long standing. Immunity is the body's way of responding to any infection and helps prevent a second infection with that germ. This is a normal part of childhood and most infants and toddlers and preschool children will have three to five such infections each year. One way to look at this is that, by exposing your child to infection, daycare actually helps your child develop her/his immune system, potentially benefiting their overall health in years to come.

The goal of this book is to provide parents with a current and easy-to-read reference on infections and the best infection control practices for children in daycare and preschool. This book provides:

- an overview of how germs are spread;
- an overview of how antibiotics should be used;
- recommendations on what to look for when choosing a daycare center or preschool for your child (e.g., specific policies on enrollment requirements, staff education, and employee health);
- guidelines for children at greater risk of becoming infected and/or developing more severe disease (e.g., infants, immunocompromised children, and children with congenital and chronic diseases);
- recommendations for what a center should do if an outbreak occurs at the facility; and
- information on specific germs with detailed information on:
  ○ who carries the germ,
  ○ how the germ is spread,
  ○ how long the incubation period lasts,
  ○ how long an infected child can transmit the germ, and
  ○ the management of the illness, including prevention, recommended number of days out of daycare, and recommended care.

Not all of my experience with childhood infections has been professional. As a young mother, after a long day working at the hospital caring for very sick children, I would pick up my two sons at daycare before heading home. I will never forget the one evening when I arrived in the midst of story time. I happily settled myself on a tiny chair against the wall of the classroom to listen along with the eight healthy children seated around their loving, dynamic teacher.

But then my quiet respite was shattered.

The teacher pulled a hankie from inside her blouse and proceeded to wipe all of their runny noses with the one piece of cloth.

As a result, I dedicated my first book to my sons. The goal of that first book was to provide practical guidance on infection control for pediatricians, family practitioners, nurse practitioners, public health professionals, child care providers, and preschool teachers.

Now, my sons are married. This new book is dedicated to my grandsons and intended to help all of the mothers and fathers who ask these questions:

- Is my child too sick to go to daycare today?
- When can my child, who is getting over an infectious illness, return to daycare?
- What should I look for in a daycare center to ensure that my child will be safe, happy, and healthy?

Leigh B. Grossman, MD
Charlottesville, Virginia

ACKNOWLEDGMENTS

I would firstly like to acknowledge the authors who not only provided their expertise, time, and scholarship in writing this book, but who, as respected colleagues and pediatricians, have spent their lives treating and preventing the spread of infection in children.

I would like to thank the parents who provided the worries and the questions that have kept me writing and focused on this book.

Anne Carley, of Chenille Books, is the newest addition to my "wing men and women." She has provided the wisdom, experience, and roadmap to move a manuscript into published book form. I am sincerely grateful and in awe of her kind guidance and phenomenal expertise and know that she is a quiet jewel in this arena.

I owe David Morris immense gratitude for his author advice and for his incredible tutoring, mentoring, wisdom, coaching, nudges, and applause. One could not have a better teacher and friend!

To Darcey Lacy at Watermark Design and her team of artists and visual scripters who have pushed me from the academic to the trade format with creativity and patient guidance, I am beyond grateful.

I wish to thank my assistant Dianne Shifflett, who single-handedly organized, edited, and provided the secretarial assistance that makes this book as good as it is.

I wish to thank my sons Nick and Jeff, who were the original daycare children for whom this book was written. They and their wives Julia and Kate have provided the best expertise, advice, critique, and unwavering support. My grandsons Brock and Taylor are now repeating the cycle, keeping me current and focused on the new generation of daycare kids and what we all want their daycare and preschool worlds to be.

Leigh B. Grossman, MD

INTRODUCTION

With the vast majority of U.S. parents working full time while raising children, the need for daycare has exploded in recent decades. As a result, the opportunities to transfer viruses, bacteria, and even parasites from one child to others in close contact are frequent, with important implications for those infected, the daycare personnel who have responsibilities to limit transmissions, and the parents and grandparents who transport the children to and from their homes. All are at risk for these infections.

Most of the infections are short lived and mild, and an important part of developing a normal immune system, but occasionally more severe infections arise with adverse outcomes. It is important to minimize these more threatening transmissions. Several infections that arise in daycare settings are preventable through vaccination; however, in an era of distrust of many national institutions, an active anti-vaccine movement has challenged public health authorities and physicians, putting daycare centers and families at risk because of a lack of immunity.

Leigh Grossman is a nationally recognized pediatric infectious diseases physician with insightful views of their epidemiology. In this remarkable volume, she has assembled a team of experts who offer critical perspectives useful for parents who have or soon will have children in daycare.

For specific infections, the chapters are organized into signs and symptoms, cause, spread and control, and the diagnosis and treatment. The accessible language and clear advice make this a very readable book.

On a personal note, Leigh is a former fellow, a friend, and colleague. It is a special honor to have seen her career rise to such distinction. This is the greatest gift of teaching. *The Parent's Survival Guide to Daycare Infections* will be a lasting tribute to her many talents.

Richard P. Wenzel MD, MSc
Professor of Infectious Disease and
  Former Chairman, Internal Medicine
Virginia Commonwealth University
Richmond, Virginia

PART I

INFECTION ESSENTIALS

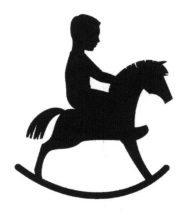

Tommy & the Stomach Bug

Tommy is three years old. When his mother picks him up from daycare, he says that he had a fun day, he ate his lunch, and he had a nap. His mom buckles him into his car seat and they head home.

En route, the car is quiet and when his mom checks the rearview mirror, Tommy is sound asleep. Twenty minutes later, she arrives home, unstraps the little man who doesn't want to walk into the house (he usually runs!) and she notices he is warmer than usual.

As they settle in at home and she begins to prepare dinner, Tommy is on the sofa, quiet, and stating that he has a stomach ache. He has, on closer look, red cheeks, a rash on his little belly and back, and he soon develops diarrhea and vomiting. What Tommy has, his mom learns at the pediatrician's that night, is a "stomach bug," a gastrointestinal infection caused by a virus that is known to be going around at his daycare center.

Tommy's mother and the doctor discuss what this means. How did Tommy get it? He "caught this" from close contact with the other children, touching toys or objects contaminated by other children, or from caregivers who are carrying the germ.

How do you prevent his getting such a virus in the daycare setting? This is almost impossible, given that the children are like puppies crawling over each other, touching, playing, using the same tables, mats, chairs, toys, and surfaces all day.

What is the good news? This illness usually lasts only two to three days, leaves no lingering effects in the otherwise healthy child, and provides them with immunity that protects them from getting sick when they encounter this germ again.
Part I of this book, Infection Essentials, introduces the five major types of infections, and how germs, including viruses like Tommy's, are spread in daycare and preschool.

1

WHAT IS AN INFECTION?

Leigh B. Grossman

An infection can be asymptomatic (without any symptoms) or symptomatic, can be of short duration, chronic (of long duration) and/or lifelong depending on the patient and the specific germ. There are five major groups of living organisms that can cause infection.

Bacteria ▶ Bacteria are ubiquitous and live everywhere in our environment, on us, and in us, and mostly do not cause infection and may even be protective. Examples of bacteria that are common causes of disease include streptococci (sore throat), pertussis (whooping cough), and salmonella (diarrhea).

Viruses ▶ Viruses are infectious agents that can multiply only when they are inside other living host cells. Once the virus finds a susceptible host, it multiplies and can cause disease such as influenza (the flu), herpes simplex (fever blisters), rotavirus (gastroenteritis), and rhinovirus (common cold).

Fungi ▶ Fungi are germs that include molds, yeast, and mushrooms. These organisms are ubiquitous in nature and rarely cause disease. Examples of fungal infections are candida (diaper rash and thrush), *Tinea pedis* (athletes foot), and *Tinea corporis* (ringworm).

Protozoa ▶ Protozoa are living organisms that are ubiquitous in nature and are often spread via contaminated water. Examples of protozoa that cause disease are giardia (gastroenteritis) and amebae (gastroenteritis).

Parasites ▶ Infections caused by parasites include head lice and worms.

The common signs and symptoms of childhood infections are well known to all parents. The specific diseases that these particular signs and symptoms may suggest are detailed below.

1.1   Common Signs and Symptoms of Childhood Infection

Coughing	Respiratory infections, bronchiolitis, sinusitis, pneumonia caused by respiratory syncytial virus, parainfluenza, influenza, adenovirus, pertussis, *Haemophilus influenzae*, pneumococcus, and others
Diarrhea	Multiple infectious agents including salmonella, shigella, campylobacter, yersinia, giardia, cryptosporidium, rotavirus, enterovirus, and parasites
Fever	May be a general symptom of viral or bacterial diseases
Headache and/or stiff neck	May be a symptom of many illnesses but with fever may represent bacterial or viral meningitis
Infected skin or sores	May represent impetigo, herpetic infection, chickenpox, or wound infection, and child should not be allowed in daycare without physician consent
Irritability that is unusual, or unexplained crying	May be a symptom of many illnesses but with fever may represent bacterial or viral meningitis
Itching of body or scalp	Close observation for lesions or agents such as scabies or lice
Lethargy	May be a general symptom of viral or bacterial diseases

1.1 Common Signs and Symptoms of Childhood Infection (continued)

Pink eye	Tearing, itching of eye, swelling, and tenderness, along with redness and/or discharge from the eye represents conjunctivitis, either viral or bacterial in nature
Rapid or altered breathing	Respiratory infections (See Coughing, above)
Rash	Generally must be evaluated on a case-by-case basis; whenever there is a question as to the cause, physician should be consulted
Sore throat	Respiratory infections, pharyngitis, tonsillitis, viruses, and group A streptococcus (strep throat)
Stomatitis (mouth sores)	May be a symptom of viral gingivostomatitis (coxsackie, herpes)
Vomiting	May be a general symptom of viral or bacterial diseases
Yellow skin and/or eyes	May be a symptom of hepatitis, and child should not be allowed in daycare without physician consent

2

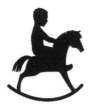

HOW GERMS ARE SPREAD

Jeffrey R. Donowitz

Daycare centers and preschools provide a unique setting conducive to the spread of germs. Preschool aged children who are susceptible to virtually every infection congregate daily with their peers. Each child brings viruses, bacteria, and parasites from his or her own family to share.

The gathered children have habits of personal hygiene that are either questionable (at best) or deplorable (on average). A child who acquires an infection may generously share these germs with adult workers in the daycare center, with peers at the center, and/or with his or her own parents and siblings at home.

This book would not be needed if we had an easy and practical method to prevent transmission of germs in the daycare or preschool environment. Although there is no foolproof method to prevent transmission, understanding how infectious agents move from one person to another is the first step toward limiting their spread via common sense interventions such as hand-washing.

Three steps are required for transmission of an infectious agent from an infected individual to an uninfected person. First, the germ must be excreted by the infected person from a site such as the nose or the mouth or in the feces. Excretion does not occur through the skin (except from boils, impetigo, or varicella) or through clothes. Second, the excreted germ must be transferred to the well person. Transfer could be through the air (aerosol spread), by direct contact (hand-holding), or by way of an intermediary surface (door knobs). Finally, the infecting agent must reach a susceptible site (usually the mouth, the nose, or the eye) to infect the well person. It is important to understand that different pathogens utilize different modes of spread and different points of entry. Generally, a respiratory pathogen on the skin of a well person does not infect that person unless it is inoculated onto a susceptible mucosal surface (such as the nose or eye).

The sites from which organisms are excreted by an infected child are known. Agents (viruses, bacteria, and parasites) that infect the gastrointestinal tract are excreted in the feces. Viruses and bacteria that infect the respiratory tract are excreted in respiratory tract secretions (nasal mucus, droplets in cough or sneezes) and not in feces. Cytomegalovirus is excreted in both saliva and urine. Quick Reference 2.1 details where organisms are excreted.

The three transmission steps are detailed in Quick Reference 2.2 and may be illustrated with three examples. In the first, transmission of a virus causing gastroenteritis (such as rotavirus) would begin with excretion of the virus in the diarrheal stool of the sick child. Transfer to a well person would result from fecal contamination of the hands of the person while changing the diaper of the infant. It could also occur via a well person touching a contaminated surface such as a changing table. The final step, inoculation of a susceptible site, requires that the well individual put his or her hands or contaminated articles into his or her mouth. The virus, after being swallowed, would then infect the lower gastrointestinal tract. Transmission by this fecal–oral route could be interrupted by removing the contaminating virus from the hands of the individual by the use of soap and water.

The second example is provided by transmission of a bacteria that causes gastroenteritis (such as salmonella) and begins with eating or drinking contaminated food or water. Food (such as chicken) is often contaminated and remains infectious if undercooked. Water contamination is often from a contaminated source such as a fouled well. The bacteria are unknowingly ingested. Prior to ingestion they can be spread via hands, contaminated counter tops, utensils, or dishes to a well person who then moves the bacteria from the contaminated surface to their mouth.

A third example is provided by transmission of respiratory viruses (rhinovirus, respiratory syncytial virus), which are excreted in nasal secretions and may be in droplets expelled during coughing or sneezing. Different viruses utilize different human functions such as the cough, sneeze, or runny nose to maximize their spread. Viruses in droplets may be transferred to the well person by way of the air. Susceptible mucosal sites would be inoculated as the well person breathes the droplet-contaminated air. The frequency of transmission of agents through the air is probably small, although this is not known for certain. On the other hand, viruses in nasal secretions may contaminate the hands of the sick person and articles in the environment by way of the hands. Transfer to the hands of the well person occurs during contact with contaminated articles or the hands and nasal secretions of the sick child. Inoculation, the final step in transmission, requires that the hands of the well person contact the lining of his or her own nose, mouth, or eye so as to deposit the virus on the mucosa. This self-inoculation step could be interrupted by handwashing before mucosal contact, such as occurs from nose or eye rubbing.

What can be done to prevent transfer of infectious pathogens in the childcare setting? Constant cleaning of the diaper changing area is an obvious means of reducing environmental contamination with fecal material. Careful handling, preparation, and storage of food and water are imperative for the prevention of food and waterborne infection. Frequent handwashing by adults working in the childcare center is one control measure that all could agree is needed to prevent both self-inoculation and transfer of pathogens contaminating hands to other children. Teaching children correct handwashing techniques and hygienic practices, as age appropriate, is also crucial to the prevention of pathogen spread. The availability of handwashing facilities and the importance of the repetitive use of these facilities by children and personnel cannot be overemphasized.

2.1 How Germs Are Spread in the Daycare Center or Preschool

	Bacteria	Viruses	Parasites
Direct	Group A streptococci *Staphylococcus aureus*	Herpes simplex Herpes zoster *Molluscum contagiosum*	Pediculosis Scabies
Respiratory	*Bordetella pertussis* Group A streptococci *Haemophilus influenzae* *Mycobacterium tuberculosis* *Neisseria meningitidis*	Adenovirus Influenza Measles Parainfluenza Respiratory syncytial virus Rhinovirus Varicella	
Fecal–oral	*Campylobacter* *Escherichia coli* *Salmonella* *Shigella*	Enteroviruses Hepatitis A Hepatitis E Rotavirus Calicivirus Astrovirus	*Cryptosporidium* *Giardia lamblia* Pinworms
Contact with infected blood and secretions (urine, saliva)		Cytomegalovirus Hepatitis B Hepatitis C Herpes simplex Human immunodeficiency virus	

2.2 Three Steps Required for Transmission of an Infectious Agent[a] from an Infected to an Uninfected Person

Excretion	Pathogen must be excreted from site(s) by infected person
Transfer	Pathogen must be transferred to well person
Inoculation	Pathogen must reach susceptible site in well person

---

[a] Infectious agent could be bacteria, viruses, or parasites.

PART II

BEST PRACTICES: INFECTION CONTROL POLICIES THE DAYCARE CENTER OR PRESCHOOL SHOULD FOLLOW

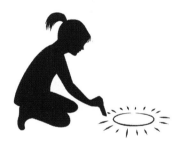

Dana, Dave, & Daycare

Dana and Dave are expecting their first baby. Dana is a radiology technician at the local hospital and Dave is a computer programmer working for one of the large insurance companies. They know that between the two of them, they will do all they can to keep their infant at home with one of them for the first two months.

They are eager to secure daycare options and placement for their infant after they both return to full-time work. Their choices are a small, unregulated daycare home, or a large daycare center that is a franchised chain. They know that having a nanny at home is financially prohibitive.

As they interview and tour their options, they realize that this is a world they do not know. What should they be looking for, what do they want for their baby, and what questions should they ask?

New parents like Dana and Dave need to read Part II of this book, which details the infectious disease standards that parents should expect at the facility they choose for their children and, most specifically, their infants. We look at best practices for daycare centers and preschools for preventing and controlling the spread of infections that are common in this setting. These practices and procedures should be available in writing for the parents to review.

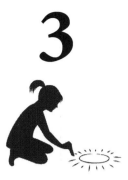

3

PREVENTING INFECTION: RECOMMENDED POLICIES FOR THE CENTER, ATTENDEES, AND PERSONNEL

Terry Yamauchi

RECOMMENDED POLICIES FOR THE DAYCARE CENTER OR PRESCHOOL

Liaison with Parents and Physicians ▶ Daycare and preschool staff can be a very important resource for the health promotion and maintenance of the children they care for. It is important that they maintain a close working relationship with parents and physicians to ensure that enrollee and staff vaccinations are up to date and health problems are promptly identified and adequately managed. Parents should be notified of community and in-facility exposures to infectious diseases. Transition times with parents at the beginning and end of the day should be used thoughtfully. Parents should be asked to identify symptoms of infection in the child or household members at drop-off time and the staff should alert parents to any concerns in their child at the end of each day.

Liaison with Public Health ▶ Daycare and preschool staff should maintain a close working relationship with their local public health departments. Daycare staff should understand that the public health department in their local community is responsible for all children as opposed to the parents' primary concern for their own child and the physician's primary concern for his or her patient. Centers should be networking with other healthcare providers and other childcare centers. This is particularly important during periods of seasonal illnesses such as influenza and other respiratory infections.

Physical Organization ▶ There should be separate rooms and caregivers for diapered and nondiapered children. Food preparation areas must be separate from diaper change areas; each area should have separate handwashing facilities. Bathrooms must include handwashing facilities. Cribs should be separated by at least 3 feet to decrease the transmission of airborne pathogens, and bedding and mattresses should not be shared unless thoroughly cleaned between users.

Staffing Issues ▶ A staff:child ratio of 1:3 or 1:4 and a small group size (8 to 12 infants maximum) are recommended. Staff require training and ongoing supervision of their work. Assignment of a primary caregiver for each child will reduce exposures and thus the risk of infection. Responsibilities for diaper changing and food and formula preparation should be assigned to different staff as much as possible. Infants should also be protected from other children and caregivers who are ill with colds or other infections. Handwashing and personal hygiene of all staff should be stressed.

ATTENDEE POLICIES

Children attending daycare or preschool should be free of known infections unless the center has specific and separate facilities dedicated to the care of the sick child. Behavioral characteristics of the preschool child make for easy transmission of infectious agents. Because of the difficulty in identifying contagious illnesses during the incubation period and the well-known fact that infection may be present and transmissible well before symptoms develop, it is imperative that when an infection is recognized, alternative childcare be arranged. Parents or guardians should be carefully questioned as to symptoms of infection in the attendee as well as other family members (siblings and parents). Symptoms such as fever, lethargy, poor feeding, decreased activity, or unusual behavior should be a warning that the onset of illness may be occurring. Although these symptoms do not necessarily warrant exclusion from the childcare facility, close observation for further developing illness is indicated.

Alternate Care for the Sick Child ► Symptoms such as fever, diarrhea, vomiting, rash, skin lesions, wound infections, cough, or runny nose should alert parents and personnel to the strong likelihood of an infectious disease. The symptoms listed above may also be the result of other conditions not related to infectious agents; however, most often they are associated with transmissible infectious organisms, and whenever possible another care source for these children should be sought. On enrollment, the parent needs to provide the alternate arrangements to be made when a child is identified as ill during the day. Parents must understand the center's policies on ill children and the exclusion guidelines set out by public health authorities.

Attendee Immunizations ► Daycare and preschool attendees should be up-to-date on their immunizations. The following vaccines are highly recommended for children attending daycare and preschool: diphtheria, *Haemophilus influenzae* type b, hepatitis A, hepatitis B, influenza, mumps, pertussis, pneumococcus, polio, rotavirus, rubella (German measles), rubeola (measles), tetanus, and varicella (chickenpox) (Quick Reference 3.1). These recommendations are only meant to be a guide. The choice of immunizing agent should be at the discretion of your child's doctor. Stronger or different recommendations may be made during outbreaks and/or epidemic situations. In some states, mandatory immunizations are required for attendance in schools and daycare facilities. Check with state health authorities for required immunizations.

Attendee Medical History ► Every effort should be made to obtain a full medical history on all children attending the center. Essential medical information should include immunization records, known allergies, past illnesses, infections, trauma, and medications. Any child from a high-risk setting should be screened for tuberculosis prior to enrollment.

PERSONNEL POLICIES

Daycare and preschool personnel should be medically screened prior to hire, be free of known and transmissible infections, and understand the requirement to maintain high standards of personal hygiene. A medical history should be obtained from the daycare employee. The history should recognize employee susceptibility by documenting previous infections, immunizations, and medications. Especially important is the history of childhood illnesses such as measles, mumps, rubella, and chickenpox to determine the childcare workers' current immune status to the vaccine-preventable diseases. This information takes on added importance in that the immunity induced by some vaccines appears to lessen over a period of time (e.g., pertussis and measles vaccines); other vaccines do provide lifelong protection, and the protected and unprotected employee should be identified. Specific immunization recommendations for daycare and preschool personnel are outlined below. (Quick Reference 3.2)

Personnel taking medications that suppress the immune response may be at increased risk for infections. Although corticosteroids are the medications more frequently associated with decreasing the immune response, the usual dosage for acute treatment (i.e., allergic reactions) may not be a high enough dose to compromise the normal host response. Even long term corticosteroid therapy for such diseases as asthma or systemic lupus erythematosus may not suppress the normal host response enough to cause concern. Higher doses of corticosteroids or chemotherapeutic agents used in cancer and/or transplant patients are the conditions that place the daycare worker at significantly increased risk of infection and then transmitting that infection to other children. If there is any question regarding the employee's immune status, the daycare center should require a statement clarifying the current status from his or her prescribing physician. As stated above, the employee should be free of known and transmissible infections and maintain high standards of personal hygiene.

Tobacco use, if allowed, should be restricted to areas away from children.

Preemployment Physical Examination ► A physical examination should be obtained to ensure that personnel are physically able to carry out the tasks assigned for the area of employment. Obvious physical disorders that may be conducive to transmission of infectious diseases, such as dermatitis, must be cleared by a physician before the employee is allowed to work in areas of child contact. Daycare workers should be screened for tuberculosis prior to employment.

Preemployment Culturing of Personnel ► Culturing for gastrointestinal pathogens is still required in some states, and individual state health regulations should be reviewed. In general, culturing of daycare personnel before employment is of little value and should not be necessary. However, personnel should be informed that culturing may be required during an outbreak investigation.

Personnel Immunizations ► The following vaccines are highly recommended for daycare and preschool employees: diphtheria, hepatitis A, hepatitis B, influenza, meningococcus, mumps, pertussis, pneumococcus, polio, rubella (German measles), rubeola (measles), tetanus, and varicella zoster (chickenpox-herpes zoster) (Quick Reference 3.2).

Diphtheria–tetanus toxoid vaccines have been widely used in the United States and have markedly decreased the incidence of these diseases. Because of the seriousness of these two diseases and the fact that childcare workers may be at higher risk, diphtheria–tetanus toxoid vaccination should be carried out every 10 years. It may be necessary to reimmunize personnel who have wounds thought to be contaminated and if more than 5 years have lapsed since the vaccines were last administered.

Rubeola (measles), mumps, rubella (German measles), and varicella (chickenpox) vaccines are live, attenuated viruses. Although live vaccines, there is little evidence to prove that they pose any risk of infection to an immunized adult or child. Daycare personnel lacking a history of disease or immunity (antibody) by laboratory testing (if available) should receive the vaccines.

Poliomyelitis is a disease that has almost disappeared in the United States, and this accurately reflects the value of the poliovirus vaccines. The inactivated poliomyelitis vaccine (IPV) is currently the recommended vaccine for childhood immunization in the United States. It is advised that daycare and preschool personnel be fully immunized against poliovirus. The inactivated poliovirus vaccine is the vaccine of choice for the unvaccinated childcare worker.

The current drop-off in use of the pertussis vaccine for infants has resulted in an increase in whooping cough in infants and children. Speculation has also been raised as to the increased susceptibility of previously immunized adults. In 1994, adolescents and older individuals were found to be the second largest group (after infants) to contract pertussis. Transmission of whooping cough from infants and children to adult caretakers and family members has been demonstrated. Of perhaps greater concern is the transmission of the bacteria from the adult caretaker to the unprotected infant or child. Reimmunization of adults with the acellular pertussis vaccine has been shown to boost protection to pertussis without risk for adverse events. The acellular pertussis vaccine has been found to be effective in boosting protection to pertussis without increased risk for adverse events when administered with diphtheria and tetanus vaccines.

Influenza virus infections are well known in the daycare facility. There are two types of influenza vaccines, a killed and a live, attenuated virus. Both are recommended for daycare personnel. The live, attenuated vaccine is not recommended for individuals over 50 years of age. Unfortunately, the influenza virus undergoes periodic changes, and if those changes occur after the vaccine strains have been selected for vaccine production, the vaccine may not be protective. Since the influenza virus vaccine induces protective antibodies with a relatively short life, yearly immunization is necessary for maximum protection. Because the immune response to the vaccine requires about 2 weeks for antibody levels to become protective, in times of epidemics it may be necessary to prophylactically administer an antiviral agent if the employee has been exposed and has not been immunized.

The hepatitis A vaccine is effective and safe and should be used for all daycare workers. Although this illness is generally mild or even asymptomatic in children, it can easily spread in this setting, and the adult disease can be severe, debilitating, and prolonged.

Hepatitis B virus vaccine is recommended for all childcare workers, but, most importantly, for staff who care for those with cognitive disabilities and staff who care for children from high-risk families.

The varicella vaccine should be administered to all nonimmune childcare workers. This is a live, attenuated (not disease-causing) vaccine that may produce a few atypical pox lesions but is effective and safe in adults with normal immune function who we know will be exposed to this pathogen in the daycare setting.

The zoster vaccine is recommended for all adults over age 60.

The meningococcal vaccine is useful in the control of meningococcal disease and is recommended for all daycare workers.

The pneumococcal vaccine is recommended for the daycare worker aged 65 years or older.

PET AND ANIMAL POLICIES

Pets and animals may be advocated for use in some daycare settings. The benefit of these programs remains to be demonstrated. In many states, it is illegal to bring animals other than service dogs into facilities involved in daycare. It is advisable that the daycare facility remain in compliance with federal and state licensure regulations.

Remember that pets may be vehicles for diseases. They may initiate allergic reactions in some children, they may cause accidents, unpleasant odors may result, and they may infringe on other children's rights. Animals brought into a strange new environment may not act as they normally do in more familiar surroundings.

The list of diseases associated with pets and animals is extensive. There are many microorganisms, including bacteria, viruses, fungi, protozoa, and parasites, associated with animals commonly used as pets. With this background information, daycare centers and preschools considering the use of pets or other animals within the facility must carefully weigh the potential benefits against the potential risks of exposure of each and every individual (child and staff) within the facility. Until further information is available, it seems prudent to limit the area in which and the extent to which pets and animals can be used in a center.

RECOMMENDED CLEANING AND DISINFECTION

The child in daycare is frequently one who crawls and explores the environment with his or her mouth. Likewise, many daycare children are incontinent of urine and feces. For these reasons it is important that the environment be kept as clean as possible. Because of the increased numbers of children and the higher ratio of children to adults in the daycare setting, when compared to in the home, it may be more difficult to maintain cleanliness.

Regularly scheduled environmental cleaning, such as disinfection, vacuuming, sweeping, dusting, and washing, is an essential element of preventing the spread of infectious agents. Standard household cleaning materials are adequate for most environmental surfaces. Care should be taken to ensure proper dilutions and removal after use because of the potential toxicity of many standard products.

Special care may be needed in certain locations such as food preparation and consumption, diaper changing, toilet, and sleep areas, as these are higher in risk for transmission of infectious agents.

Contaminated Surfaces ▶ Special cleaning of contaminated surfaces requires removal of organic material, followed by the application of a commercial cleansing agent. With the concern over acquired immune deficiency syndrome (AIDS) caused by the human immune deficiency virus, additional precautions are indicated. Blood and body fluids contaminated with blood (blood is visible) should be flooded with a bleach solution diluted 1 part bleach to 10 parts water. Many commercial cleansing agents are also acceptable for this purpose, but the label should be carefully reviewed for this use. After thorough soaking, the mixture (contaminated material plus cleansing agent or bleach solution) should be carefully removed, and the area cleaned with the routine product.

Bedding ▶ Individual bedding should not be shared and must be washed at least weekly.

Carpets ▶ Carpets are special surfaces that are extremely difficult to maintain. In general, the same principles apply, but because carpeting may remain wet for long periods of time and thus retain infectious material, the drying of the carpet following cleanup, as for other surfaces described above, is imperative. Previously contaminated carpets are of high risk for transmitting infectious agents, even if cleaned, until they have dried.

Toys and Play Equipment ▶ In the childcare setting, toys and play equipment may be shared by many children, and the potential for transmitting infections is obvious. Toys are especially challenging because of the varying materials and textures involved. In general, soft, cuddly toys should be discouraged, as they require washing and drying, which may be much more difficult than toys of impervious materials. Infants may play with washable toys that are disinfected before and after use by another infant. To clean, wash toys with dishwashing detergent and water, then rinse in a dilute (1:10 to 1:100) bleach solution. Infants should not be given shared, nonwashable soft toys that may be contaminated with infectious secretions.

HANDWASHING PROCEDURES

The importance of handwashing cannot be taken lightly. Hand transmission of infectious agents has been recognized for more than 100 years. Handwashing is the single most important procedure for preventing the transmission of infections in the daycare and preschool setting. For example, a 50 percent reduction in diarrhea cases was observed in centers adopting a careful handwashing regimen.

Handwashing is the mechanical removal of infectious agents. In the daycare center, soap and water are all that is needed to carry out this procedure. What must be taught and reinforced is the importance of performing handwashing correctly and frequently.

Daycare employees should be taught that handwashing prevents the employees from infecting themselves or their family members, as well as protects the children in their care.

For routine handwashing, the hands should be vigorously rubbed together for at least 10 seconds with enough soap and water to lather all surfaces. Thorough rinsing and drying should follow. Liquid soap is preferable. If bar soap is used, it should be stored in a manner to allow complete drainage of water.

Handwashing should be carried out when visible contamination or soiling occurs, after use of the toilet, following diaper changes, after handling any body fluids, before and after eating or feeding, and after tending children with known infections.

To facilitate correct, frequent handwashing, a sink, running water, soap, and clean, preferably disposable, dry towels are necessary.

DIAPERING PROCEDURES

Since so many children in the daycare setting are not toilet-trained, diaper changes are necessary. Correct changing of diapers is required to prevent the spread of infectious agents in the fecal material. Even asymptomatic children may harbor infectious microorganisms in their stools. Spread of diseases via the fecal–oral route is well documented but can be prevented when proper procedure is followed.

It is essential that the diapering area is separated from areas of food preparation and feeding. Disposable diapers are the preferred materials. Cloth diapers may be stored with the paper diapers, but both should be kept far from the area of the soiled diapers to prevent contamination. The changing surface should be away from other child activities and covered with a smooth, moisture-resistant, cleanable cover.

A tightly covered container with a foot-operated lid is preferred for the soiled diapers. A plastic trash bag or disposable container should be placed into the plastic container. This must be emptied and cleaned daily, or more frequently as needed.

When changing the soiled diaper, disposable gloves may be used if so desired or available. The removed soiled diaper should be folded inward to cover fecal material. The child's skin is then cleansed to remove stool. Soap and water may be needed to remove visible soiling. After the clean diaper has been applied and the child has been removed from the changing area, the soiled diaper is placed in the covered container. The changing surface is cleansed with a detergent spray or soap and water and allowed to dry. Hands of the child and caregiver must be carefully washed whether gloves are used or not.

FOOD PREPARATION

Food preparation areas require sinks and towel supplies separate from diaper change facilities. Hands must be washed before food and formula preparation and before feeding an infant. Food should be refrigerated, and any unused food or formula discarded within 24 hours.

Quick References begin on next page.

3.1 Recommended Vaccines for Daycare Center and Preschool Attendees

Vaccine	Comment
Diphtheria (killed)	Immunization at 2, 4, 6, and 18 months of age, repeated at school entry and every 10 years throughout life
Haemophilus influenzae type b conjugate (killed)	Immunization at 2, 4, 6, and 15 months of age
Hepatitis A (killed)	Two doses 6 to 12 months apart, starting at 12 months of age
Hepatitis B (killed)	Immunization at birth, 1, and 6 months of age
Influenza (killed or live, attenuated)	Yearly immunization for all children 6 months of age and older. Children who received no doses of monovalent vaccine the previous season require two doses of the current influenza vaccine
Meningococcus (killed)	Immunization after 2 years of age
Mumps (live, attenuated)	Immunization at 15 months of age, repeated at 4 to 6 years of age
Pertussis, acellular (killed)	Immunization at 2, 4, 6, and 18 months of age, repeated at school entry and every 10 years throughout life
Pneumococcus (killed)	Immunization at 2, 4, 6, and 12 to 15 months of age
Polio (killed)	Immunization at 2, 4, and 18 months of age, repeated at 4 to 6 years of age
Rubella (live, attenuated)	Immunization at 15 months of age, repeated at 4 to 6 years of age
Rubeola (live, attenuated)	Immunization at 15 months of age, repeated at 4 to 6 years of age
Rotavirus (live, attenuated)	Immunization at 2, 4, and 6 months of age
Tetanus (killed)	Immunization at 2, 4, 6, and 18 months of age, repeated at school entry and every 10 years throughout life
Varicella (live, attenuated)	Immunization at 12 to 18 months of age

3.2 Recommended Vaccines for Daycare Center and Preschool Staff

Vaccine	Comment
Diphtheria (killed)	Booster every 10 years
Hepatitis A (killed)	Proof of immunization or disease in the past
Hepatitis B (killed)	Proof of immunization or disease in the past
Influenza (killed or live, attenuated)	Yearly
Meningococcus (killed)	Proof of immunization
Mumps (live, attenuated)	Proof of immunization or disease in the past
Pertussis, acellular (killed)	Booster every 10 years
Pneumococcus (killed)	For adults over age 65
Polio (inactivated)	Proof of immunization
Rubella (live, attenuated)	Proof of immunization or disease in the past
Rubeola (live, attenuated)	Proof of immunization or disease in the past
Tetanus (killed)	Booster every 10 years
Varicella (live, attenuated)	Proof of immunization or disease in the past
Zoster (live, attenuated)	For adults over age 60

3.3 Questions to Ask when Choosing a Daycare Center or Preschool

General Policies

☐ Are there separate rooms and caregivers for diapered and nondiapered children?

☐ Are food preparation and feeding areas separate from diaper change areas?

☐ Are proper handwashing procedures and personal hygiene for staff stressed?

☐ How often are the center, bedding, toys, and play equipment cleaned?

☐ When must children stay home because of illness?

☐ How are parents notified of illnesses among children?

☐ Does the center have a "sick room" for children with minor illnesses?

☐ Does the center keep a record of health-related problems, such as illnesses, injuries, and accidents, for each child?

Attendees Policies

☐ Is a physical examination required before admission?

☐ Are children required to have certain vaccinations before coming to daycare?

Personnel Policies

☐ Is a medical history required of staff prior to hire?

☐ Is a physical examination required of staff prior to hire?

☐ Are staff required to have certain vaccinations prior to hire?

Pet and Animal Policies

☐ Are animals present at the center? If yes, what policies are in place to prevent the spread of infection and to maintain safety?

4

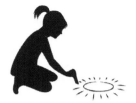

TREATING INFECTION: APPROPRIATE AND INAPPROPRIATE ANTIBIOTIC USE

Leigh B. Grossman

Excessive and inappropriate use of antibiotics has been a source of concern almost since their introduction into the practice of medicine in the late 1940s. As these medications achieved easy availability and widespread use, the problem became ever more acute, to the extent that by the early 1990s, children in this country were receiving an average of one oral antibiotic prescription per year, in many cases for the treatment of self-limited viral upper respiratory infections. For example, in a recent study of pediatric office visits, it was found that an antibiotic was prescribed for almost half of children with a common cold and 75 percent of those with "bronchitis," conditions for which antibiotics offer no benefit. Although the unwarranted use of antibiotics for acute respiratory tract infections has been reduced by more than a third in the last decade, over-prescribing of antibiotics continues to be prevalent and remains a major public health concern.

The reasons for over-prescribing are multiple and can be laid at the feet of parents, health care providers, managed care organizations, and even daycare centers and schools. Parents may, given their need to return their child to some form of daycare as soon as possible, request antibiotic treatment, "just to be on the safe side," even if told it will be ineffective. In many cases, both parents have employment outside the home, making the need to send their child to a daycare center or preschool both imperative and urgent. These facilities in turn, provide additional impetus for demanding antibiotics by policies that call for any "sick" child to be on antibiotic treatment before being allowed to return. Finally, health care providers, cognizant of these perceived needs, intent on keeping parental approval and managed care endorsement, respond to the pressure and acquiesce to these demands.

The public health consequences of these behaviors are profound. It has been stated that antibiotics are unique in the sense that, unlike other medications, treatment of an individual can affect an entire community. Thus, the use of antibiotics will, after a relatively short period of time and sometimes after only a single dose, select out antibiotic-resistant bacteria for survival in the upper respiratory tract. These antibiotic-resistant organisms can then be spread readily via unwashed hands or respiratory secretions to any close contacts: siblings, parents, playmates, and daycare center and preschool personnel. They, in turn, can pass these resistant bacteria on to their contacts. Because resistant organisms tend to die out after several months and are replaced by antibiotic-susceptible bacteria, this problem is not permanent. However, every time a child receives an antibiotic, the potential for reinstituting the cycle begins once again. When the exposed community is a daycare center or preschool, each child on unnecessary antibiotic treatment represents a potential threat to all children attending that facility. When the facilities require antibiotic treatment as a criterion for the return of a sick child, they are, in a sense, perpetuating a situation that, under more conservative policies, would resolve on its own.

How does injudicious use of antibiotics affect the community, particularly the childhood community? The adverse effects of antibiotics can have direct consequences for the individual receiving them. It has been estimated that up to ten percent of persons taking an antibiotic medication will experience at least one side effect. These are usually relatively minor and can include allergic rash, abdominal pain, diarrhea, nausea and vomiting, vaginal or skin yeast infection, and far less frequent but more serious reactions such as anaphylactic or allergic shock, hemolytic anemia, life-threatening vasculitis, and hepatitis. Notably, any of the more common reactions can require home care, often for several days, negating the presumed advantages of treating, "just to be on the safe side."

Of no less importance are the indirect effects engendered by the acquisition and transmission of antibiotic-resistant bacteria. When children who carry these organisms in their nose and throat acquire an ear infection, sinusitis, or pneumonia, treatment with standard primary therapy will often fail, resulting in a delay in appropriate treatment, prolongation of illness, possibly more severe infection, and the need for additional therapy with an antibiotic possessing a broader spectrum of action, with higher cost and generally more side effects. At the present time, between 15 and 40 percent of pneumococci in the United States are resistant to amoxicillin, the antibiotic generally recommended for first-line therapy of otitis media and sinusitis, two of the most common pediatric bacterial upper respiratory infections caused by this organism. One strain has recently been shown to be resistant to all FDA-approved and several investigative antibiotics. In contrast, in Holland, where antibiotic use is voluntarily restricted by practitioners, the incidence of pneumococcal amoxicillin resistance is around 2 to 5 percent. Among many of the organisms considered in other chapters in this book, antibiotic resistance has been a considerable problem. Thus, in addition to pneumococcal infection, those caused by staphylococci, streptococci, meningococci, *Haemophilus influenzae*, salmonella, shigella, gonococci, and tuberculosis are all likely to be due to an antibiotic-resistant organism.

APPROPRIATE ANTIBIOTIC USE FOR SPECIFIC UPPER RESPIRATORY TRACT INFECTIONS

Ear Infections ▶ The clinical manifestations of an ear infection include fever, irritability, sleep disturbance, poor appetite, and pulling at the ear in preverbal infants. Older children may complain of ear pain, difficulty hearing, and vertigo. Sometimes, pus or bloody discharge from the ear is present. Fever occurs in one-third to two-thirds of children with ear infections. Acute otitis media is often preceded by a viral cold with runny nose and cough.

Most infections are caused by a germ called the pneumococcus. The other major causative agents are *H. influenzae* (nontypeable strains), *Moraxella catarrhalis*, and group A streptococcus (particularly during the winter).

The diagnosis of an ear infection is made with a history of rapidly (usually less than 48 hours) progressing signs and symptoms together with an ear examination. Pain alone is never a sufficient criterion to make this diagnosis. Discomfort felt in the ear can be caused by numerous conditions other than an acute ear infection, including tonsillitis, a blocked eustachian tube, fluid in the ear (otitis media with effusion), infection or foreign body in the ear canal, or infection of the soft tissues and structures around the ear (mumps parotitis, lymphadenitis, dental abscess).

Antibiotics are generally recommended for persistent signs and symptoms of an ear infection. Recent recommendations encourage an "observation option" with pain medication but no antibiotics for 48 hours for children over 2 years of age who are not toxic or experiencing severe pain. Clinical worsening or failure of resolution by the end of that time warrants antibiotic therapy. It is estimated that 80 percent to more than 90 percent of ear infections will resolve without antibiotic therapy. Pain (acetaminophen, ibuprofen, codeine) and fever (acetaminophen, ibuprofen) control is an essential part of treatment.

Influenza vaccine can be effective in preventing ear infections during the influenza season. Pneumococcal vaccine can prevent about 6 percent of all ear infections and 20 percent of recurrent (defined as equal to or more than 5 per year) ear infections. Ear infections are not contagious, and exclusion from daycare or preschool is only required until the child is free of fever and is able to participate in general activities. No special precautions are required for other children at the center, personnel, or family.

The Common Cold ▶ The clinical manifestations of the common cold are stuffy nose, runny nose, cough, sore throat, fatigue, and poor appetite. Less frequently, children complain of headaches, muscle aches, fever, and chills. A viral infection of the eye (conjunctivitis, pink eye) sometimes accompanies the respiratory symptoms. Signs and symptoms of a cold may persist or even worsen for the first few days, but gradually improve thereafter.

Typically, nasal discharge with an uncomplicated viral cold will proceed over the first week from a thin, watery discharge to a cloudy discharge, a yellow-green discharge, and then slowly resolve. Appearance of a yellow-green discharge does not indicate the presence of a secondary bacterial infection. Of those children who cough and have a runny nose with a cold, 50 percent may still be coughing and 25 percent may still be complaining of nasal stuffiness at 14 days of illness. Thus, the common cold is often a 2- to 3-week illness.

Ear infection may occur during the first week of a cold with additional symptoms, particularly in infants and young children. Persistent and unimproving nasal discharge and daytime cough for 14 days or longer suggests the presence of acute bacterial sinusitis. Children with asthma may experience worsening of their reactive airways disease with upper respiratory infections.

The germs causing the common cold are the rhinovirus, coronavirus, parainfluenza virus, and respiratory syncytial virus. Less often, influenza virus, metapneumovirus, adenovirus, and enterovirus cause the common cold.

The diagnosis is usually based on clinical signs and symptoms and a history of contact with another infected person.

Antibiotic therapy is not indicated, and no specific therapy is available. Saline nasal irrigation and aspiration of nasal mucus with an ear-bulb syringe for infants, limited use of sympathomimetic nasal sprays (neosynephrine, oxymetazoline) in older children, and antipyretics and analgesics (acetaminophen, ibuprofen) can provide symptomatic relief. Placing young infants in an infant seat can help with drainage of nasal secretions.

The infectious period varies with the causative agent, but generally is during the time that nasal secretions are present.

Influenza vaccine and pneumococcal vaccine may be effective in preventing ear infections during the respiratory season. Exclusion from daycare or preschool should only be until the child is free of fever and able to participate in general activities. Transmission to other children, personnel, and families is largely via fingers contaminated with viruses from toys, countertops, and other environmental surfaces and can be reduced by frequent handwashing, careful secretion/excretion control, and making certain that tissues are discarded in a closed container.

Cough Illness/Bronchitis ▶ The early clinical signs and symptoms are those of the common cold, but within a few days the cough becomes more prominent, dry at first and then productive or "wet." Fever is common the first 5 to 7 days. Mild substernal (below the breastbone) chest pain is not uncommon in older children during the early phases of the illness. Children with asthma may experience worsening of symptoms. The causative germs of cough illness/bronchitis are generally the same as those of the common cold. The diagnosis is based on signs and symptoms and a history of contact with infected people. Unimproving daytime cough lasting more than 14 days may represent acute bacterial sinusitis.

Antibiotic therapy is not indicated, and no specific therapy is available. Children over 48 months of age with a dry, nonproductive cough experiencing gagging or sleep difficulty may be given an antitussive medication such as dextromethorphan (DM). Children between 12 and 48 months of age may obtain relief from their cough with the use of one or two teaspoons of honey given every 4 to 6 hours. Honey should not be used in children under 12 months of age because of the risk of infantile botulism. Any cough medicine should be used with caution in all children with a productive "wet" cough and/or asthma. Antipyretics and analgesics (acetaminophen, ibuprofen) can provide symptomatic relief.

The infectious period varies with the etiologic agent, but is generally during the first week or two of cough. Other than influenza vaccine, no vaccine is available for prevention. Children should be excluded from daycare or preschool until they are free of fever and able to participate in general activities without disruption of classes due to cough. Transmission to other children, personnel, and families can be reduced by frequent handwashing and disposal of tissues in a closed container.

Acute Bacterial Sinusitis ▶ The common cold is considered a viral rhinosinusitis; bacterial sinusitis is a complication identified by the severity of the illness or the persistence of symptoms. Thus, clinical manifestations include either a "severe" or "persistent" form: "Severe" acute sinusitis presents with high fever, an ill appearance, facial pain, and mucopurulent nasal discharge. The "persistent" form is far more common and presents as 14 or more days of unimproving nasal discharge of any quality together with a daytime cough (which may be worse at night). Appearance of a yellow-green nasal discharge during the first week of a common cold does not indicate the presence of acute bacterial sinusitis.

The etiologic agents that cause bacterial sinusitis are the same as those causing ear infections. The diagnosis of sinusitis is based on clinical findings, which are adequate in almost all cases to establish a diagnosis. Radiographs to confirm or rule out the presence of bacterial sinusitis in children 6 years of age or younger are not recommended. Although they may be useful in older children, they are rarely indicated.

Antibiotics are always indicated for the "severe" form of acute sinusitis and at 14 or more days of "persistent" sinusitis symptoms. Additional treatment such as that recommended for symptoms of the common cold and cough illness/bronchitis is appropriate when indicated.

Acute bacterial sinusitis is not contagious. Influenza vaccine and pneumococcal vaccine may be effective in preventing acute bacterial sinusitis during the respiratory virus season. Exclusion from daycare or preschool is recommended until the child is free of fever and able to participate in general activities. There are no recommendations or special precautions for other children, personnel, or families.

Sore Throat (Pharyngitis) ▶ The clinical manifestations of pharyngitis in infants and young children often include a refusal to eat, irritability, and sleep disturbances. Older children complain of sore throat and, when there are large and/or painful inflamed lymph nodes in the neck, they may complain of associated neck pain. Viral pharyngitis is often part of a common cold and accompanied by one or more of the following: rhinitis, cough, hoarseness, rash of the throat called an enanthem, conjunctivitis, or diarrhea. Presence of any of these signs is strong evidence against a "strep throat." The throat and tonsils may look normal, slightly red, or intensely red with an exudate. Fever is usually low grade and brief in duration. The pain of pharyngitis can be referred to the ear, leading to confusion with acute otitis media. The presence of an exudate does not always indicate group A streptococcal (GAS) infection.

Streptococcal sore throat is usually rapid in onset and can be accompanied by headache, abdominal pain, enlarged and tender lymph nodes below the jaw, and significant fever (≥102°F). A red, papular "sandpaper" rash on the body may accompany the pharyngitis (scarlet fever). The throat is usually red and swollen. Tonsillar infection with pus (exudate) and small red spots on the palate (palatal petechiae) may or may not be present but, when present, are suggestive but not diagnostic of GAS infection.

The causes of a sore throat include viruses, which represent about 80 percent of all sore throats and are caused by the same organisms as those responsible for the common cold. GAS is the most common germ causing a sore throat.

The diagnosis of a streptococcal sore throat is made with throat culture or a rapid detection test. Diagnosis based on clinical appearance of the throat is highly unreliable.

No specific treatment is available for viral pharyngitis. Antibiotic therapy is indicated for treatment of laboratory proven streptococcal sore throat.

Quick Reference begins on next page.

4.1 A Guide to Judicious Antibiotic Use

- Recognize that most childhood upper respiratory infections are caused by viruses. Your daycare center or preschool should not require that children with "a cold," "sore throat," "hoarseness," "cough," or "snotty nose" be on antibiotics or excluded from attendance.

- Recognize that the average normal infant and young child may have as many as 5 to 10 viral upper respiratory infections a year, most during the winter, each lasting from 1 to 3 weeks. Thus, having a viral cold for much of the winter would not be abnormal or unusual. The larger the daycare center or preschool, the greater the number of contacts with infected children and the greater the number of such infections.

- Utilize the guidelines provided in chapters 6 and 7 to educate yourself on appropriate policies for treatment, exclusion, and return.

- Make sure your center and caregivers abide by the recommended guidelines.

- Recognize that most childhood upper respiratory tract bacterial infections can be treated at home with therapies that are administered once or twice a day. Children on antibiotics should be permitted to attend daycare or preschool if they are free of fever and able to participate in general activities.

- If your child requires antibiotic therapy during childcare hours, provide caregivers with:
  - Clear instructions regarding storage (including storage temperature), administration, and duration of therapy.
  - A graduated syringe or dosage cup; teaspoons or tablespoons should not be used, as their volume varies widely.
  - A masking substance (e.g., chocolate syrup, marmalade, preserves, jelly) to facilitate acceptance of bad-tasting medication.

5

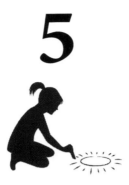

CONTROLLING INFECTIONS: ISOLATED AND EPIDEMIC ILLNESS

Leigh B. Grossman

An estimated 12 million children under 5 years of age in the United States are enrolled in part and full time regularly scheduled childcare. These infants and young children are particularly susceptible to many infectious agents due to their limited immunity, the degree of close contact between children and staff, and the lack of hygienic practices amongst this population. Infectious diseases readily spread among the children, staff, family members, and community. The childcare setting carries a great potential for infectious disease outbreaks.

An outbreak or epidemic is defined as a recent or sudden excess of cases of a specific disease or clinical symptom. Individual cases of certain diseases, such as measles, constitute an outbreak. A foodborne outbreak occurs when two or more persons experience gastrointestinal tract disease after ingesting the same food or water.

The investigation of an outbreak or suspected outbreak of a disease is usually not required for every infectious problem identified. In some situations, the factors associated with the problem may be obvious and the daycare center can readily implement control measures without conducting an investigation.

However, if the factors (causative agent, source, and/or mode of transmission) associated with the problem are unknown or if additional cases occur despite the institution of control measures, the daycare or preschool should conduct a systematic investigation of the outbreak (Quick Reference 5.1).

EPIDEMIC INVESTIGATION

What the Daycare or Preschool Center Should Do ► To verify a reported or suspected infectious disease in a child, contact the child's physician. The local health department may be contacted to assist in the investigation as well as follow-up of exposed persons. After the diagnosis is confirmed, a decision to proceed with the investigation depends on multiple factors such as causative germ, immune status of the children and staff exposed, mode of transmission, incubation period of the infectious disease, and the time interval between onset of the illness in the first case and notification of the center.

If the illness is causing severe disease or death, the problem is unique or unusual, or there is a possibility of litigation or political pressure, the problem should be investigated. If the problem has occurred previously or the center understands the contributing factors, they should immediately implement infection control measures without an investigation.

After the diagnosis is confirmed, immediate infection control measures to contain or interrupt the transmission of the infectious disease should be implemented. Parents and all members of the daycare setting should be informed of the outbreak and implementation of these control measures (Quick Reference 5.2). More specific control measures may be necessary as more information becomes available during the investigation.

The nature of the case or infectious problem that is occurring should be defined in order to recognize existing or new cases. The definition should be based on the causative germ, site of infection, and/or clinical signs and symptoms. As the investigation proceeds, further information may be obtained that will require the case definition to be revised.

The search for existing and new cases is necessary in order to estimate the magnitude of the problem. All parents and daycare or preschool staff should be educated regarding signs and symptoms of the illness so they can monitor exposed children and staff for the onset of the illness.

What Parents Should Do ▸ Families should be asked to notify the center if their child becomes ill. All absences should be documented for time and reason.

EPIDEMIC HYPOTHESIS

Based on the data collected, a tentative hypothesis or an educated guess as to the causative germ, the source of infection, and the likely mode of transmission of the infectious disease should be formulated. This hypothesis should explain the majority of cases and permit intervention and control measures to be instituted. Unless an outbreak is associated with a commercial product, severe disease, or death, and if the outbreak clears with the institution of infection control measures, there is no need for further intervention.

The final step in the investigation of an outbreak is a written summary of the findings and recommendations to prevent a similar occurrence in the future. The completed report should be disseminated to management and the individuals involved in the investigation.

EPIDEMIC PREVENTION

As detailed in the previous chapters, to prevent the spread of communicable illness among children and staff, health policies must be designed to reduce the risks associated with infections in the daycare setting. In addition, the daycare or preschool administrator should be observant of illnesses occurring in staff and participants to determine whether patterns of infections occur. If a pattern is detected, prompt intervention is necessary. A resource consultant (e.g., public health provider, pediatrician) should be available to assist the daycare center or preschool in determining appropriate measures to prevent the spread of infectious diseases.

5.1 Systematic Approach to Outbreak Investigation

Formal investigation should:

- Verify the diagnosis of the reported or suspected case (illness).
- Implement interim infection control measures.
- Develop a case definition.
- Search for existing and new cases.
- Characterize the cause by person, place, time, and risk factors.
- Formulate a tentative hypothesis.
- Update infection control measures.
- Test the hypothesis. (In most daycare centers or preschools, this step may be eliminated unless resources are available to conduct the necessary studies.)
- Write a report summarizing the results of the investigation.
- Inform parents of findings, resolution, and what preventive measures have been instituted.

5.2 Examples of Interim Epidemic Control Measures

Your childcare center should:

- Notify all families of the increased incidence of an illness or illnesses at the center.
- Wash hands with soap and water immediately after handling infants, blowing noses, changing diapers, or using toilet facilities, and before handling food. Alcohol-based hand gels are an effective alternative if hands are not visibly covered with secretions or excretions. The use of disposable gloves is helpful but not a substitute for good hand disinfection and handwashing practices.
- Discourage sharing of personal articles and toys.
- Clean soiled surfaces with a disinfectant rated by the U.S. Environmental Protection Agency or with household bleach diluted 1 part bleach to 100 parts water.

5.2 Examples of Interim Epidemic Control Measures (continued)

- Change clothing as soon as it is soiled; place it in a plastic bag to be sent home.
- Use disposable diapers; discard into a covered container.
- Group infected or exposed children with personnel who are not caring for noninfected or unexposed children.
- Assess staff's risk and need for intervention to ensure that all employees are protected.
- Exclude new admissions to the daycare center or preschool during the outbreak.
- Notify families of all children; re-emphasize that they should keep the sick child or children at home.

PART III

IS MY CHILD TOO SICK TO GO TO DAYCARE? QUICK REFERENCES FOR SPECIFIC INFECTIONS

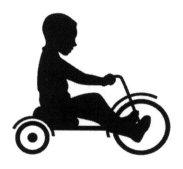

Elizabeth Doesn't Feel So Good

Brian and Susan are both professionals in Kansas City. Brian works as a trial attorney and has a big case with opening statement starting in the morning. Susan is an Emergency Medicine physician and her shift starts at 0800 hours at the local hospital.

Elizabeth, their four year old, wakes up at midnight, comes into their room and says she doesn't feel good. She has a fever of 101°. They give Elizabeth acetaminophen and everyone goes back to sleep until 5:30, when the alarms go off and their day starts. Elizabeth looks okay, but a bit droopy. She has no fever this morning, has a bit of a runny nose, and doesn't want much to eat.

Elizabeth is given more acetaminophen, taken to preschool where she happily walks into the building, and both parents take off for their busy and demanding days – with a prayer that the school doesn't call them about a returning fever and/ or increasing symptoms.

In Part III, we provide handy reference materials for the busy parent, like Brian or Susan, who needs to make a quick decision about whether to send their child to daycare in a situation like Elizabeth's. We summarize what to do when your child is diagnosed with, or exposed to, an infection. We also provide a list of symptoms to watch for when your child has been exposed to many contagious illnesses, so that you know when it's time to call the doctor.

6

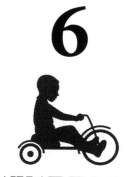

WHAT TO DO
WHEN YOUR CHILD HAS BEEN
DIAGNOSED WITH OR EXPOSED TO
AN INFECTION

Leigh B. Grossman

For each infection, listed by the common name or the biologic name of the germ, this table provides you with what secretions and excretions are infected, the incubation period during which the child may have no symptoms but is harboring the germ, and a comment column that details how long the sick child (the **Case**) or his or her family members, daycare personnel, and other daycare children (the **Contacts**) should be excluded from attendance.

Quick Reference begins on next page.

6.1 Communicable Diseases in Daycare Centers and Preschools

Infection	Infective Material	Incubation Period	Comments
Amebiasis (Entamoeba histolytica)	Feces	2–4 weeks	*Case:* Exclude during acute illness, until treated and until stools are free of oocysts.
			Contacts: Exclude symptomatic contacts until stools are screened for oocysts.
Campylobacter enteritis	Feces Contaminated food or water	1–7 days	*Case:* Exclude until 48 hours of effective therapy or until asymptomatic, whichever is shorter.
			Contacts: Exclusion not required.
Chickenpox (varicella)	Infected exudate Respiratory secretions	10–21 days	*Case:* Exclude until lesions are dry and crusted.
			Contacts: Exclude immunosuppressed children during outbreak.
Conjunctivitis			
—Bacterial	Purulent exudate	24–72 hours	*Case:* Exclude until 24 hours of effective therapy.
			Contacts: Exclusion not required.
—Viral (adenovirus, etc.)	Purulent exudate	12–72 hours	*Case:* Exclude until exudate resolves.
			Contacts: Exclusion not required.

Infection	Infective Material	Incubation Period	Comments
Cytomegalovirus	Infected urine and saliva	1 month	*Case:* Exclusion not required.
			Contacts: Exclusion not required.
Diarrhea	Feces	1–3 days	*Case:* Exclude until symptoms resolve.
			Contacts: Exclusion not required.
Escherichia coli O157:H7	Feces Contaminated food	2–6 days (usually 3–4 days)	*Case:* Exclude until two serial stool cultures negative or until 10 days after cessation of symptoms.
			Contacts: Stool cultures not indicated in absence of symptoms.
Fifth disease (erythema infectiosum, parvovirus B19)	Respiratory secretions	4–14 days (usually 12–14 days)	*Case:* Exclusion not required.
			Contacts: Exclusion not required.
German measles (rubella)	Respiratory secretions	14–21 days (usually 16–18 days)	*Case:* Exclude for 7 days after onset of rash.
			Contacts: Those who are pregnant and not immunized should seek medical advice.
Giardia lamblia	Feces Contaminated food or water	1–4 weeks	*Case:* Exclude until asymptomatic.
			Contacts: Exclusion not required.

Infection	Infective Material	Incubation Period	Comments
Gingivostomatitis (herpes simplex virus)	Infected secretions	3–5 days	Case: Exclude until cutaneous lesions are dry and crusted.
			Contacts: Exclusion not required.
Haemophilus influenzae	Respiratory secretions	2–14 days	Case: Exclude during acute illness and until treated.
			Contacts: Seek physician's advice concerning prophylaxis.
Hand, foot, and mouth syndrome (Coxsackie A16)	Feces Respiratory secretions	4–6 days	Case: Exclusion not required.
			Contacts: Exclusion not required.
Hepatitis A	Feces	15–50 days (usually 20–30 days)	Case: Exclude until 10 days after onset of symptoms and symptomatically able to participate in general activity.
			Contacts: Prophylaxis should be considered for staff and children.
Hepatitis B	Infected saliva or blood	6 weeks–6 months	Case: Exclude during acute illness and children with chronic hepatitis B surface antigens who bite or cannot contain secretions.
			Contacts: Exclusion not required.

Infection	Infective Material	Incubation Period	Comments
Impetigo contagiosa (Staphylococcus)	Lesion secretions	7–10 days	*Case:* Exclude for 48 hours of effective therapy.
			Contacts: Exclusion not required.
Infectious mononucleosis	Saliva	5–7 days	*Case:* Exclude until symptomatically able to tolerate general activity.
			Contacts: Exclusion not required.
Influenza	Respiratory secretions	1–3 days	*Case:* Exclude until symptomatically able to tolerate general activity.
			Contacts: No exclusion required. Seek physician's advice concerning prophylaxis and immunization.
Lice (pediculosis)	Infested area	Approximately 7–10 days after eggs hatch	*Case:* Exclude until treated.
			Contacts: Examine for infestation and recommend treatment if needed.
Measles (rubeola)	Respiratory secretions	6–21 days (usually 10–12 days)	*Case:* Exclude until 5 days after appearance of rash.
			Contacts: Check immunization status. Exclude immediately on signs of illness.

Infection	Infective Material	Incubation Period	Comments
Meningitis —Meningococcal	Respiratory secretions	2–10 days	*Case:* Exclude during acute illness and until treated.
			Contacts: Seek physician's advice concerning prophylaxis and immunization.
Mumps (infectious parotitis)	Respiratory secretions	12–25 days	*Case:* Exclude for 9 days from onset of swelling; less if swelling subsides.
			Contacts: Susceptible contacts should seek physician's advice.
Pharyngitis (sore throat)			
—Nonspecific	Respiratory secretions	12–72 hours	*Case:* Exclude only if child has fever or is unable to participate in general activities.
			Contacts: Exclusion not required.
—Streptococcal	Respiratory secretions	1–4 days	*Case:* Exclude for 24 hours of effective therapy.
			Contacts: Exclusion not required.
Pinworms (*Enterobius vermicularis*)	Feces, contaminated surfaces, clothing, bedding, towels, etc.	2 weeks–2 months	*Case:* Exclude until treated.
			Contacts: Exclusion not required.

Infection	Infective Material	Incubation Period	Comments
Pneumococcal infections (otitis media, respiratory infections, meningitis, bacteremia)	Respiratory secretions	Varies with type of infection (1–30 days)	*Case:* Exclude only if child has fever or is unable to participate in general activities.
			Contacts: Exclusion is not required. Susceptible contacts should seek physician's advice concerning immunization.
Respiratory infections (upper respiratory infections, colds, bronchitis)	Respiratory secretions	12–72 hours	*Case:* Exclude only if child has fever or is unable to participate in general activities.
			Contacts: Exclusion not required.
Roseola	Probably respiratory secretions	5–15 days	*Case:* Exclude until rash has disappeared.
			Contacts: Exclusion not required.
Rotavirus	Feces	1–3 days	*Case:* Exclude until asymptomatic.
			Contacts: Exclusion not required.
Salmonellosis	Feces Contaminated food	6–72 hours	*Case:* Exclude during acute illness, usually 5–7 days.
			Contacts: Stool cultures not indicated in absence of symptoms.

Infection	Infective Material	Incubation Period	Comments
Scabies	Infested areas	2–6 weeks; 1–4 days after reinfestation	Case: Exclude until treated.
			Contacts: Direct inspection of body.
Scarlet fever (Streptococcus)	Respiratory secretions	1–4 days	Case: Exclude for 24 hours of effective therapy.
			Contacts: Exclusion not required.
Shigellosis	Feces	1–7 days (usually 1–2 days)	Case: Exclude for 5 days of antibiotics or until stool cultures are negative.
			Contacts: Stool cultures indicated only in suspected outbreak.
Tuberculosis	Respiratory secretions	2–10 weeks	Case: Exclude until physician advises return.
			Contacts: Seek physician's advice concerning prophylactic treatment.
Whooping cough (pertussis)	Respiratory secretions	Respiratory secretions 7–21 days (usually 7–10 days)	Case: Exclude until 5–7 days of effective therapy and physician advises return.
			Contacts: Seek physician's advice concerning prophylactic treatment.
Yersiniosis	Feces Contaminated food or water	2–11 days (usually 3–7 days)	Case: Exclude during acute illness.
			Contacts: Exclusion not required.

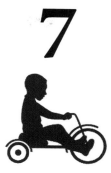

7

SYMPTOMS TO WATCH FOR WHEN YOUR CHILD HAS BEEN EXPOSED TO AN INFECTION

Leigh B. Grossman

If your child has been exposed to one of the diseases below, you may want to call your physician if any of the described symptoms appear. Better protection for all results when ill children are kept home until they have recovered.

Amebiasis *(Entamoeba histolytica)* ▶ Usually asymptomatic but occasionally varies from acute diarrhea with fever, chills, and bloody or mucoid diarrhea to mild abdominal discomfort with diarrhea containing blood or mucus, alternating with periods of constipation or remission. The incubation period is 2 to 4 weeks. The child will not be allowed to attend if the diarrhea contains blood or pus or is accompanied by fever. The child may return following treatment for the acute illness, and when stools are free of cysts.

Chickenpox (varicella) ▶ Small water blisters on the scalp, neck, and covered parts of the body are usually the first signs noted. The blisters break easily. The child may become cross, tire easily, and have a fever during the first few days of disease. The incubation period is 10 to 21 days; commonly, 13 to 17 days. Sick children must be kept at home until all lesions are dry and crusted. Consult your physician for antiviral and/or antibody therapy if your child is immunocompromised.

Conjunctivitis (pink eye) ► Inflammation of the eye, causing redness, tearing, and occasionally formation of pus. The incubation period is 12 to 72 hours for viral infection and 24 to 72 hours for bacterial infection. Children with conjunctivitis must be kept at home until 24 hours after initiation of effective bacterial therapy or, in viral disease, until purulent discharge disappears.

Cytomegalovirus ► Rarely produces symptomatic disease; when it does, it is characterized by fever, sore throat, and swollen lymph nodes (glands). The incubation period is 1 month. Children will be allowed to attend as long as they are able to function within the normal activities of their class.

Diarrhea ► Increase of frequency and change of consistency in bowel movements from the child's normal pattern; fever may or may not be present. The incubation period depends on the causative agent (salmonellosis—6 to 72 hours; shigellosis—1 to 7 days; yersiniosis—2 to 11 days; *Campylobacter*—1 to 7 days; *E. coli* O157:H7—3 to 8 days; viral—24 to 48 hours). The child will not be allowed to attend if diarrhea is accompanied by fever or other symptoms, such as vomiting, irritability, dehydration, lethargy, blood, or pus. The child may return once the diarrhea is manageable and/or symptomatic infection has been treated.

Fifth Disease (Erythema infectiosum) ► A rose-red rash (slapped-face appearance) on the face, which fades and recurs and may spread to the limbs and trunk. By the time the rash appears, the child is no longer contagious and may return to daycare or preschool.

German measles (rubella) ► A light rash, mild symptoms, with glands behind the ears and neck enlarged. The incubation period usually is 14 to 21 days. Sick children must be kept at home for a minimum of 7 days after the onset of rash and until all symptoms have disappeared.

Giardiasis ► May be associated with a variety of intestinal symptoms, such as chronic diarrhea, abdominal cramps, bloating, frequent loose and pale greasy stools, fatigue, and weight loss. The incubation period is 1 to 4 weeks. Sick children must be kept at home until diarrhea has resolved.

Gingivostomatitis (herpes simplex virus fever blisters) ► Infection may be mild to severe and is marked by fever and malaise lasting a week, accompanied by vesicular lesions in and around the mouth and nose. The incubation period is 3 to 5 days. Children must remain at home until the lesions are dry and crusted.

Hand, foot, and mouth syndrome (Coxsackie A16) ► Characterized by sudden onset of fever, sore throat, and lesions that may occur on the inside of the mouth (cheeks, gums, and sides of tongue) as well as on the palms, fingers, and soles. Occasionally, lesions appear on the buttocks. The incubation period is 4 to 6 days. Children will be allowed to attend, as long as they are able to function within the normal activities of their class, including outdoor activities.

Hepatitis A ► Sudden onset of fever, malaise, loss of appetite, nausea, and abdominal discomfort followed by jaundice (yellowing of the skin and eyes). The incubation period is 15 to 50 days. Sick children must be kept at home until physician advises return. Consult your physician for prophylactic protection of your child. Your physician may recommend hepatitis A immunization as part of a community-wide outbreak control program.

Hepatitis B ► Characterized by loss of appetite, abdominal discomfort, nausea, and vomiting. Joint pain and rash may occur as well as jaundice and a mild fever. The incubation period is 6 weeks to 6 months. Sick children must be kept at home during acute illness, and children with chronic disease who bite or cannot contain secretions will be excluded.

Impetigo ► Starts with multiple skin lesions, usually around the face and mouth and other exposed areas, such as the elbows, legs, and knees. The lesions vary in size and shape and begin as blisters but rapidly change to yellow crusted areas on a reddened base. The incubation period is 1 to 10 days. Children must remain home until they have received at least 48 hours of effective antibiotic therapy.

Infectious mononucleosis ▶ An acute syndrome characterized by fever, sore throat, weakness, and enlarged lymph nodes (glands), especially in the neck. The incubation period is 5 to 7 weeks. Child must be kept at home until symptoms disappear and he or she is able to tolerate general activity.

Influenza ▶ An acute illness characterized by fever, chills, headache, muscle aches, mild sore throat, and cough. The incubation period is 1 to 3 days. Sick children must be kept at home until general activity is tolerated. Aspirin or aspirin-containing products should be avoided during influenza infection because of the association with Reye's syndrome. Consult your physician for advice concerning prophylaxis and immunization.

Lice (pediculosis) ▶ Severe itching and scratching of the scalp. Eggs of head lice (nits attached to hairs) are small round gray lumps. Children with head lice should remain at home until they have been treated. Advise examination of household and other close personal contacts, with concurrent treatment as indicated. Clothing, bedding, and other vehicles of transmission should be treated by laundering in hot water, by dry cleaning, or by application of an effective chemical insecticide.

Measles (rubeola) ▶ Runny nose, sneezing, coughing, watery eyes, and fever, with a red blotchy rash appearing on the third to seventh day. The incubation period is 6 to 21 days; commonly, 10 to 12 days. Sick children are to be kept home for a minimum of 5 days from the appearance of the rash. Consult your physician for prophylactic protection of household contacts who have not had measles or who have not been immunized against measles.

Meningitis ▶ Meningococcal meningitis is characterized by sudden onset of fever, intense headache, nausea and often vomiting, stiff neck, and frequently a rash. The incubation period varies from 2 to 10 days; commonly, 3 to 4 days. Consult your physician regarding immunization and/or prophylactic treatment of your child.

Haemophilus influenzae meningitis has a sudden onset of fever, vomiting, lethargy, and stiff neck and back. Progressive stupor and coma are common. The incubation period is 2 to 14 days. Consult your physician regarding prophylactic treatment of your child.

Mumps (parotitis) ► Fever with swelling and tenderness in front of and below the ear or under the jaw. The incubation period is 12 to 25 days. Sick children must be kept home until the swelling of all glands involved and all symptoms have disappeared.

Respiratory infection (nonspecific) ► Runny nose, sneezing, increased tearing, sore throat, and malaise lasting 2 to 7 days. The incubation period is usually 12 to 72 hours. Child will be allowed to attend, as long as he or she has no fever and is able to function within the normal activities of the class, including outdoor activities.

Roseola ► Characterized by sudden fever, sometimes as high as 106°F (41°C), which lasts 3 to 5 days. A rash appears on the chest and abdomen with moderate involvement of the face and extremities as the temperature returns to normal. Rash lasts 1 to 2 days. Child may return to school when rash disappears.

Rotavirus ► Sporadic severe diarrhea and vomiting, often with dehydration. The child will not be allowed to attend until he or she is asymptomatic.

Scabies ► Begins as itchy raised areas or burrows around finger webs, wrists, elbows, armpits, and the belt line. Extensive scratching often occurs, especially at night, with secondary sores. The incubation period is 2 to 6 weeks; 1 to 4 days after repeat exposure. Children with scabies should be kept at home until they have been treated.

Streptococcal infections (sore throat or scarlet fever) ► Sudden illness with vomiting, fever, sore throat, and headache. Usually within 24 hours, a bright red rash appears. Some cases may not have a rash. The incubation period is 1 to 3 days. If your child has any of these symptoms, you should contact your physician. Sick children are to be kept at home until 24 hours after starting effective antibiotic therapy with clinical improvement.

Tuberculosis ► Fatigue, fever, and weight loss may occur early, while cough, chest pain, hoarseness, and coughing up blood may occur in more advanced disease. The incubation period is 2 to 10 weeks. Consult your physician regarding prophylactic treatment of your child.

Whooping cough (pertussis) ► A persistent cough that later comes in spells and may have an associated whoop. Coughing may cause vomiting. Many cases have persistent cough but never whoop. The incubation period is 7 to 21 days. Sick children should be kept at home until 5 to 7 days after initiation of effective antibiotic therapy with clinical improvement. Consult your physician regarding prophylactic treatment of your child.

Worms ► Worms passed in the stool or, occasionally, from the mouth or nose may be accompanied by wheezing, coughing, fever, diarrhea, abdominal pain, or itching around the rectum. The incubation period is about 2 months after ingestion of the worm eggs. Sick children must be kept at home until all symptoms have disappeared.

PART IV

RECOMMENDATIONS FOR YOUR HIGH-RISK CHILD

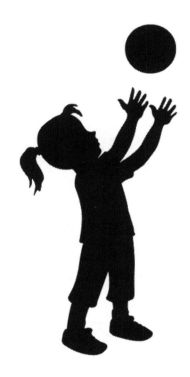

ANDY'S HEART

Andy is two, and has a very small hole in his heart that connects the two pumping chambers. The hole used to be bigger and was much more significant when he was tiny, but it is closing on its own so his parents, Ben and Mary, have been advised to watch and wait, and to work to minimize his exposure to respiratory infections.

In the meantime, Andy has been attending a small daycare home for the past year and loves it. However, every winter the other five children at this home have coughs, colds, sinusitis, and ear infections. Andy's parents want him to socialize and be with other children, but fear that he may, as the doctors have counseled, have a harder time with respiratory infections.

What should they do?

Part IV of this book examines the concerns of the parents of children, including young infants, who are at higher risk from exposure to infections that may occur in their daycare center or preschool. Andy's parents can consult the relevant chapter and prepare their questions for Andy's doctor about possible ways to keep Andy in daycare, while protecting him from potentially life-threatening infections.

8

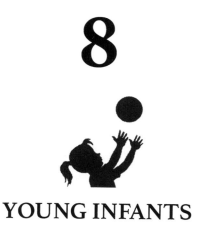

YOUNG INFANTS

David A. Kaufman

When compared with babies less than a year of age cared for at home, young infants in childcare centers are more likely to develop both minor and serious infections. In addition, signs of serious infection may be subtle. Daycare centers that care for infants must have staff who are active in health promotion and infection control practices. A young infant should be cared for by a trained, regularly assigned primary caregiver within a safe and stimulating environment. Total group size should be small, and the staff:infant ratio should be less than or equal to 1:4.

INFECTIOUS RISKS

Young infants in daycare are uniquely prone to more frequent and severe infections for several reasons.

Increased Susceptibility ▸ An infant's immune system (natural defenses against infection) is less developed and less capable than that of an older child. This results in more difficulty fighting an initial infection as well as having repeated bouts of illness with the same infectious agent.

Infants Lack Complete Immunization ▸ Infants and toddlers who have not yet received their full vaccination series are not yet protected against these preventable infections. Premature babies may also need monthly passive vaccination to protect against respiratory syncytial virus (RSV).

Increased Exposure ▶ It is normal for any child entering a group situation where exposure is increased (e.g., public school) to have more infections. Infants in group daycare face this same increased exposure from staff, other children, and even other parents. This results in ample opportunity for spreading infectious agents, primarily via unwashed hands (very common) but also through contaminated objects and surfaces.

Infants, in general, require more handling by caregivers for changing diapers, cuddling, feeding, and cleaning of facial secretions. Without proper preventive measures (e.g., hand-washing), caregivers and other children may easily transmit infectious agents from one infant to another.

Infants also have frequent hand-to-mouth contact. This increases their exposure to any infectious agents in their surrounding environment which may have been contaminated by sick staff or children or by apparently healthy children or staff who are at the beginning or end of an infectious disease. Respiratory viruses, for example, will persist for hours on surfaces. Other common infectious agents causing diarrheal illness (e.g., rotavirus, Giardia, hepatitis A, and cytomegalovirus), may live for days to weeks on toys and play mats.

Tendency to Complications ▶ While some infectious agents, such as respiratory viruses, are a nuisance when they occur in the older child, in the young infant they may lead to prolonged and/or more severe disease and complications such as ear or pulmonary infections.

COMMON INFECTIONS

Infections in infants attending daycare centers can be broken down into (1) those causing illness in infants and adults (staff, parents), such as ear, respiratory, and diarrheal infections; (2) those causing illness only in infants (e.g., *Streptococcus pneumoniae* bacteremia); (3) those causing symptomatic illness primarily in adults (e.g., hepatitis A); and (4) those causing illness only in special situations (e.g., cytomegalovirus affecting the fetus of a pregnant staff member or parent). We are all colonized with (asymptomatically carry) many common bacteria. These normal bacteria are developing increasing resistance to the commonly used antibiotics (e.g., penicillin-resistant pneumococcus, methicillin-resistant *Staphylococcus aureus*), although resulting severe infection still remains uncommon. Infants and children who attend daycare are more likely to carry antibiotic-resistant bacteria and, specifically, antibiotic-resistant *S. pneumoniae* or methicillin-resistant *S. aureus*. This emerging problem of increased incidence of antibiotic-resistant bacteria is due to both personal antibiotic use and exposure to other children who have received many antibiotics and are colonized with antibiotic-resistant organisms.

Infants are commonly and repeatedly infected with seasonal viruses, which may cause colds, diarrhea, rashes, and fevers. Colds in infants are commonly complicated by ear or eye infections and sometimes by pneumonia.

Although hepatitis A may be a common and mild infection in infants in daycare, it may cause more serious disease in susceptible adults (caregivers, parents) who are secondarily exposed at work or at home.

INFECTION CONTROL

Special Infection Control Needs ▶ In order to minimize infections and the spread of germs in this high risk group, infants do require special infection control measures that include a primary caregiver who is trained and motivated, a small group size, and a staff:infant ratio of less than or equal to 1:4.

Physical Organization ▶ There should be separate rooms and caregivers for diapered and non-diapered children. Food preparation areas must be separate from diaper change areas and each area should have its own handwashing facilities. Bathrooms must include handwashing facilities. Cribs should be separated by at least 3 feet to decrease the transmission of respiratory pathogens, and bedding and mattresses should not be shared unless thoroughly cleaned first.

Staffing ▶ A staff:infant ratio of 1:4 and a small group size with a maximum of 8 to 12 infants is recommended. Staff require training and ongoing supervision of their work. Assignment of a primary caregiver will reduce exposures and thus the risk of infection. Responsibilities for diaper changing and food and formula preparation should be assigned to different staff as much as possible. Infants should be protected from other children and caregivers who are ill.

Hand Hygiene ▶ Hand hygiene is a crucial infection control measure. The term hand hygiene has replaced the general term of "handwashing" as hands can be cleaned by either washing with liquid soap and water or by using alcohol-based hand gels. Careful handwashing dramatically reduces the transmission of infections. For example, a reduction in diarrhea rates by 50 percent was observed in centers adopting a careful hand hygiene protocol. If hands are visibly dirty or soiled, handwashing using liquid soap and water and disposable towels is required.

Diapering ▶ Hygienic precautions, especially hand hygiene, surface cleansing, and diaper disposal are required before and after each diaper change.

Food Preparation ▶ Food preparation areas require sinks and towel supplies that are physically separated from diaper changing facilities. Hands must be washed before food and formula preparation and before feeding an infant. Food, formula, and breast milk should be refrigerated and stored in individual, labeled, and lidded containers for each feeding and any unused food or formula discarded within 24 hours. Expressed breast milk should be dated and unused milk carefully labeled, refrigerated, and stored for a maximum of 72 hours.

Toys ▶ Infants may play with washable toys that are disinfected before and after use by another infant. Liquid soap and water or a nontoxic cleaning agent should be used after each use and at the end of each day. Some toys can be cleaned in a dishwasher on a daily basis using dishwasher detergent. Infants should not be given shared, nonwashable soft toys that may be contaminated with infectious secretions.

Environmental Cleaning ▶ Individual bedding must be washed at least weekly. Other surfaces should be cleaned between use or daily, depending on the item.

Surveillance of Infants for Symptoms of Infection ▶ Since signs and symptoms of infection in young infants may be subtle, primary caregivers must be watchful for any signs of infection in young infants, such as changes in feeding or behavioral patterns.

Risks to Healthy Children ▶ Healthy children exposed to infants at daycare do have an increased risk of infection. Staff working with diapered infants may directly (via hands) or indirectly (via food, mats, or toys) infect other healthy children if hygienic precautions (separate staff, separate areas, handwashing, disinfection) are not maintained. It is important to note that infected infants may appear well if they are just starting or ending an illness or have mild or clinically undetectable infections such as is the case with hepatitis A. It is therefore crucial to maintain hygienic precautions at all times. Allowing infants and older mobile children to play together increases everyone's exposure to infectious agents.

Infants who have acquired infections such as diarrhea or a head or chest cold at daycare are likely to infect 20 to 100 percent of their own healthy family members. In most cases, the healthy child, if older, will have milder disease, and the reason for separation of infants from healthy children is primarily to protect the infant. In the case of hepatitis A, infection is usually more severe in the older child or adult.

Exclusion from Daycare Center Attendance ▶ As with older children, infants should be screened daily and excluded when they have signs and symptoms of illness that require a degree of care beyond the staff's abilities and available time. The following is a list of signs and symptoms of infection in infants that should serve as attendance exclusion criteria:

- fever (rectal temperature is greater than 101°F or 38.3°C),
- rash with fever,
- diarrhea (loose stools that cannot be contained with a diaper),

- vomiting,
- unusual tiredness,
- poor feeding,
- persistent crying or irritability,
- breathing difficulties or persistent coughing, or
- yellow skin or eyes (jaundice).

When childcare staff notice any of the symptoms above, the parents should be contacted, and medical attention sought.

Recommendations for Personnel ► All personnel caring for young infants should receive specific training and ongoing supervision regarding:

- disease transmission and prevention;
- principles and practice of:
  - handwashing;
  - diapering procedures;
  - food handling, preparation, and feeding; and
  - environmental cleanliness;
- first aid and cardiopulmonary resuscitation;
- recognition of behavioral variations in both healthy and ill infants;
- maintenance of daily records on each infant, based on information from staff and parents; and
- the process for notification of other families regarding significant illness in children attending the center.

Signs of illness in young infants may be subtle. Caregivers should consistently look after the same infants and communicate closely with their parents on a daily basis so that they recognize which behaviors (e.g., feeding, temperament, stooling) are normal and which are not.

Caregivers should have written policies and procedures to deal with infant illnesses and emergencies. Ideally, daycare centers should have access to a nurse and/or physician consultant and to copies of relevant aspects of each child's current health records.

Caregivers should not look after more than three or four infants, nor should they work concurrently with toddlers and older children.

Staff who are sick with the following illnesses should not take care of infants:

- diarrhea and/or vomiting,
- measles, mumps, or rubella,
- chickenpox or shingles,
- skin infections,
- pulmonary tuberculosis,
- hepatitis,
- head colds and coughs, or
- cold sores on lips.

Parental Advice ▸ Young infants at daycare centers are prone to more frequent minor and serious infections than infants cared for at home. Exposure to and the likelihood of infection at a daycare center are dependent on:

- the total number of children at the center;
- the number of infants at the center (ideally, not more than 8 to 12 per infant room);
- the ratio of staff to infants (ideally, less than 1:4);
- the amount of antibiotic use among attendees (increased use may result in an increase in antibiotic-resistant bacteria);
- the completeness of age-appropriate immunizations for each child;
- whether or not each small group of infants has an exclusive, skilled, primary caregiver;
- the training and supervision of the staff in standard environmental infection control practices (e.g., proper handwashing after diaper changing and before food preparation and feeding);
- the floor design and availability of proper equipment to ensure safe hygienic practices (e.g., number of sinks, separate diaper and kitchen facilities, 3-foot space between cribs,

physical separation of infants and their caregivers from older children);

- protocols for environmental cleaning;
- the enforcement of specific, written exclusion policies for sick children and staff; and
- liaison with the local department of public health.

Parents must have prearranged alternative care plans for their infants in the event of illness. They should appreciate the importance and benefits of well-supervised health procedures and exclusion policies. They should always advise the daycare center of the cause of any illness necessitating their child's absence.

Parents should get to know and maintain daily communications with their child's primary caregiver.

Parents should be aware that young infants, even in excellent centers, will probably have more frequent colds and febrile illnesses, most of which will be minor. However, it may be difficult for caregivers to distinguish minor from serious febrile illnesses in infants less 6 months of age.

Parents should ensure that their children are immunized at the appropriate age with all recommended vaccines. Parents should realize that their child will be exposed to and may acquire more antibiotic-resistant bacteria and can reduce this risk by avoiding the unnecessary use of antibiotics in their own children.

9

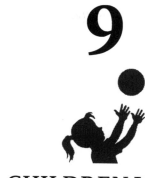

CHILDREN WITH IMMUNODEFICIENCIES

Leigh B. Grossman

INFECTIOUS RISKS

Immunodeficiencies have traditionally been divided into either those that are congenital (i.e., child is born with) or those that are acquired (after birth).

Congenital immunodeficiencies are uncommon and can affect one or more parts of the immune system. These deficiencies often become obvious shortly after birth but may sometimes become apparent only after the first few years of life. An acquired immunodeficiency refers to a deficit of the immune system that is the consequence of a disease or treatment occurring after birth. Of the acquired immunodeficiencies, the abnormalities from cancer and its treatment, transplantation and its treatment, treatment with immunosuppressive drugs, and the complications of infection with the human immuno-deficiency virus (HIV) represent the major causes of acquired immunodeficiency in childhood.

Regardless of whether the immune impairment is a defect with which the child was born or one that occurs after birth as a consequence of disease or its treatment or a new infection such as HIV, the end result is the inability to fight off germs that either are newly acquired or have already been part of the normal microbial flora.

COMMON INFECTIONS

Immunocompromised children are subject to the usual organisms that cause childhood infections (e.g., influenza, streptococci, rotavirus, respiratory synctial virus, rhinovirus, etc.). However, these fairly routine causes of childhood illness may cause more severe infection in the immunocompromised child because of their inability to contain the infection.

Additionally, the immunocompromised child may develop an invasive infection from the normal organisms colonizing their skin or mucosal surfaces (mouth, eyes, gastrointestinal tract, genitourinary system). Additionally, many of these children have indwelling vascular lines or other therapeutic devices in place and these can create their own risk for infection.

In summary, children with immunodeficiencies can become infected with a wide array of germs. Many of these organisms are part of their own normal flora and do not cause disease when the immune system is intact. Thus, for example, the child with cancer is more susceptible to infections that arise from within his or her own body than from those that occur as a consequence of exposure to others. To a large degree this is also true of children with HIV infection, although these children do have a heightened susceptibility to the common bacterial organisms that occur throughout childhood, and in particular, *S. pneumoniae* and *H. influenzae*. Although children with immunodeficiency are more vulnerable to these infections, were they to share these same organisms with children who have normal immune function, either no infection would occur, or if infection did occur, it would be no more serious than had it been acquired from a healthy child.

INFECTION CONTROL

The single overriding principle that applies to the care of immunocompromised children (as well as healthy children) is careful handwashing, especially following diaper changes or assisting with toileting procedures. Second, adherence to the principles of standard precautions when handling blood should always be followed. It is more likely that a child (or staff member) in a daycare center or preschool will not be diagnosed or recognized as being immunocompromised. Thus, staff education and adherence to simple infection control principles and procedures should be followed at all times and by everyone to keep the center safe for both children and staff members.

Special Infection Control Needs ►

- *Children with Cancer, Transplants, or Those Receiving Immunosuppressive Therapy* Since the majority of infections that arise in children who are immunocompromised because of cancer or its therapy are from organisms that are already part of those normally found in the patient's own body, they generally do not require special infection control procedures. The microorganisms responsible for causing infection in children with low white blood cell counts or in children who are receiving immunosuppressive therapy do not represent a particular hazard for children whose immune systems are normal. There are, however, some exceptions, the most notable of which are viruses such as the chickenpox-zoster virus and measles. Children with cancer or those receiving immunosuppressive therapy who have not had a prior history of chickenpox or who have not been vaccinated and are exposed to an individual with chickenpox or zoster (shingles) are at risk of developing primary chickenpox. Untreated, this infection can be extremely serious in the immunocompromised child and carries a significant risk of severe illness or even death. Fortunately, the use of antiviral therapy, if administered promptly, significantly reduces the severity of the disease and the risk of death associated with primary chickenpox in an immunosuppressed individual. As the chickenpox-zoster vaccine has become more widely used, it has also decreased the prevalence of this virus and thus, the risk of infection. Although the chickenpox-zoster vaccine is not currently recommended for use in immunocompromised children, it is anticipated that herd immunity (i.e., immunity in large numbers of children, resulting in decreased risk for infection for those who are not immunized) could decrease the overall risk for this infection. Nonetheless, the current objective is to attempt to prevent chickenpox by recognizing when an exposure has occurred and administering immunoprophylaxis to the immunosuppressed child. Thus, if there are active cases of chickenpox in the daycare center, children who are immunosuppressed should not be in attendance. When an exposure occurs in the center, the physician of the child with cancer or those receiving immunosuppressive therapy should be notified immediately. In almost all instances, the recommendation will be for the child to receive varicella-zoster immune globulin within 72 hours of exposure as this has been shown to either reduce the severity of the infection or prevent infection following exposure entirely. Similarly, children who are immunosuppressed and who are exposed to a youngster who has developed measles should also receive immunoprophylaxis with gamma globulin in order to attempt to reduce the severity of the infection or prevent the disease entirely.

For the child with cancer, two additional infection control issues apply. First, although it is acceptable for children with low blood counts to attend daycare or preschool, it must be noted that when their white blood cell count is low, they are at risk for developing an infectious complication, primarily with organisms that arise from within their own body. Fever is the major predictor of infection in patients with neutropenia. Consequently, if a child with cancer who is neutropenic becomes flushed and appears febrile or has lethargy or lassitude, his or her temperature should be taken by the oral or axillary (armpit) route. If the temperature is elevated above 38°C, the child's parents or caretakers should be notified, and most likely, the child will need to be admitted to the hospital to receive antibiotic therapy until the source of the fever is determined or the period of risk (low neutrophil count) has passed. The second specific consideration applies to children who have indwelling vascular catheters. Of course, these catheters should not be manipulated in the daycare or preschool environment, but if the child complains of tenderness around the skin or on the chest wall or along the abdomen where the catheter is placed, visual inspection to determine whether there is redness or tenderness should be undertaken. If this is the case, immediate medical attention is necessary, since an infection along the catheter site is likely. Similarly, if the child develops a fever, even in the absence of low blood counts, and has an indwelling catheter, it is important that the child's parents and physician be notified, since, again, antibiotic therapy is likely to be necessary. However, in none of these cases do the infections that arise represent hazards for other healthy children or childcare workers.

• *Children with HIV Infection* Children with HIV infection are at risk for infections that arise from both their own indigenous flora and those that can be acquired from sources outside their own body. Since the predominant bacterial infections that occur in children with HIV infection are due to bacteria with capsules such as *S. pneumoniae* or *H. influenzae*, it is quite possible that these organisms might be acquired from other children in a daycare setting. However, since these organisms are ubiquitous (common), although less prevalent as a result of the targeted vaccines, it is not reasonable to impose any particular isolation or restriction that would exclude children with HIV disease.

For both children with cancer and children with HIV infection, there are few data regarding the hazards of exposure to immunocompetent individuals who have been recently vaccinated. Although most vaccinations with attenuated (live virus that doesn't cause disease) or killed viruses or bacteria are not likely to cause problems, it is possible that excretion of certain viruses from the live virus vaccines such as oral poliovirus or chickenpox might represent a hazard for the child who is severely immunosuppressed.

Risks to Healthy Children ►

• *Children with Cancer, Transplants, or Those Receiving Immunosuppressive Therapy* The vast majority of infections that occur in children undergoing cancer therapy are with organisms that do not cause disease in the immunocompetent child. Thus, normal healthy children are not at increased risk for infection simply by having close contact with children with cancer.

• *Children with HIV Infection* Although children with HIV infection do have an increased rate of infection with common bacterial organisms such as *S. pneumoniae* and

81

H. influenzae, there are no data to support that children with HIV infection are more contagious or that the organisms are more virulent. Chronic infection with salmonella and tuberculosis are more prevalent in children with HIV and these could represent infection risks to healthy children. For salmonella, routine protocols for handwashing are imperative and HIV-infected children who are infected with salmonella should be excluded. Although the majority of mycobacterial infections that occur in children and adults with HIV infection are due to atypical organisms, tuberculosis in urban areas, particularly with drug-resistant strains, have been particularly associated with individuals infected with HIV. Although children who develop primary tuberculosis infections are usually not contagious, a child with active tuberculosis should be excluded until the infection is no longer transmissible.

Most of the fungal organisms that occur in children with HIV are not a risk for healthy children. Candida is a common organism and most normal children are already colonized with it. Cryptococcal infection occurs only rarely in children with HIV infection, and person-to-person spread with this organism does not occur. Although histoplasmosis can occur in children with HIV infection, this organism is ubiquitous in many geographic locations and the risk would not be increased by contact with children with underlying HIV infection. Similarly, most of the parasitic infections that might occur in children with HIV disease are not likely to represent infectious hazards to immunocompetent or healthy children. Gastrointestinal infections associated with cryptosporidia or *Isospora belli* can be a significant cause of diarrhea in the HIV-infected child. These organisms can cause transient infection in other immunosuppressed children as well as in children with normal immunity. However, in healthy children, symptoms are transient and chronic infection does not occur. Thus, exposure to an HIV-infected child with cryptosporidia diarrhea does not represent a hazard to the healthy child in the daycare or preschool setting.

Similar to children with cancer or those receiving immunosuppressive therapy, chickenpox can be a more significant infection in children with HIV disease. In addition, chronic or persistent cutaneous infections with the chickenpox-zoster virus can occur in HIV-infected children. If the HIV-infected child does develop active chickenpox, he or she should not be in a daycare or preschool setting until the infection has resolved. Should a healthy child acquire the chickenpox-zoster virus from an HIV-infected child, the infection will not be more serious than if it had been acquired from a healthy individual.

The major concern, of course, centers around the possible transmission of HIV itself within the daycare or preschool setting. Fortunately, this is an extremely difficult virus to transmit, and transmission can only occur by direct contact with blood or through sexual activity. Casual contact such as playing or interacting in a normal family setting is not associated with the transmission of HIV infection. Indeed, a number of studies have demonstrated that even close contact, including kissing and sharing of food and eating utensils, and other supplies, does not carry a risk for transmission of this virus. Much has been made about the possibility of transmission of HIV by biting. However, the likelihood of transmission by this route is remote. At this time, the American Academy of Pediatrics recommends that only children who engage in repetitive biting behavior be excluded from daycare or school. Thus, the only concerns that require attention for transmission of HIV should center on either blood transmission or sexual activity. Should the child with HIV infection have an injury that bleeds, or have a bloody nose, or have a cutaneous lesion that is oozing blood, care should be taken in assisting the child. The use of standard precautions is always recommended as a routine practice because it is possible that a child may be unrecognized as being infected with the HIV virus. Thus, children and staff should be educated that whenever there is a youngster or an individual who has a bleeding lesion, gloves should be worn and bloody fluids that may have spilled onto the floor, toys, or surfaces should be cleaned with a dilute (1:10 to 1:100) solution of bleach and water.

Hepatitis B virus is transmitted in a similar way to HIV but is far more contagious, presumably because the number of viral particles in blood or body fluids is much higher for the hepatitis B virus than for HIV. The most effective precautions that should be used to prevent the transmission of hepatitis B are those of standard pre-cautions and universal immunization. Thus, if standard precautions are exercised, they will be effective against both the hepatitis B virus and HIV. While hepatitis B is not found in the stool, hepatitis A can be transmitted by the fecal–oral route and underscores the importance of handwashing.

Cytomegalovirus is also a ubiquitous organism in immu-nocompromised children and can be acquired by anyone. Of most concern is transmission to a pregnant woman who has never had this infection (seronegative). Urine or secretions are the likely sources for infection and spread of infection can be prevented by scrupulous handwashing when body secretions and excretions are handled.

While precautions are easier to employ when the child is known to be infected or immunodeficient, it must be underscored that within a daycare center, it is likely that the diagnosis will be unrecognized or that information may be withheld. Thus, especially in areas of the country where the rate of HIV is highest (i.e., large urban areas), it is likely that children with undiagnosed or undocumented HIV will be found in daycare centers and preschools.

Parental Advice ► Parents should be reassured that the presence of a child who has cancer, who is receiving immunosuppressive therapy, or who has HIV does not represent a threat to the health of their child. Education is the best way to provide assurance. The now vast experience of household contacts, as well as those in various school settings, should provide reassurance that contact with children with AIDS or those who are severely immunosuppressed because of cancer treatment will not result in transmission of diseases beyond those that could be acquired from otherwise healthy children. Any time children are in a closed setting, the likelihood for transmission of a variety of common infectious diseases is increased. However, children with AIDS or those receiving immunosuppressive therapy are not more likely to transmit infection but are more likely to acquire certain types of infections. Thus, the parent of the healthy child can be reassured that his or her child will not be exposed to undue hazard by having contact with a child with cancer or with a child who has decreased immune function because of a variety of therapies or because of HIV infection.

Exclusion from Daycare or Preschool Attendance ▶

• *Children with Cancer, Transplants, or Those Receiving Immunosuppressive Therapy* The major reasons for exclusion are when the child requires medical care or has an infection that is clearly transmissible to healthy children or staff members. Relatively few infections that occur in the child with cancer or those receiving immunosuppressive therapy represent hazards to other children and thus their exclusion from attendance would include infections with the varicella-zoster virus manifested either as chickenpox or shingles or infection with the measles virus. Although the child with normal immune function who has never had chickenpox and has been exposed to an infected child is at risk to develop chickenpox 10 to 21 days after the exposure, the child with cancer or who is receiving immunosuppressive therapy has a longer period of risk that might extend up to 28 days after the infectious exposure. Thus, a child with cancer may need to be excluded from the daycare center or preschool from day 10 to 28 after an exposure if he or she is at risk to develop primary varicella. Risk is defined as a negative history of infection or a negative antibody titer against the varicella-zoster virus. Should the child have another potentially communicable disease, such as tuberculosis, exclusion from the center is necessary until the child is no longer infectious. It should be noted, however, that similar precautions would pertain to immunocompetent children who might acquire a similar infection.

• *Children with HIV Infection* Similar to the child with cancer, only rarely is it necessary to exclude the child with HIV infection from the daycare center. Indeed, the major infectious hazards that would represent a source of concern would be if the child has an infection with tuberculosis, varicella, or measles. Similar guidelines and durations of exclusion would be followed for the child with HIV infection, as was noted for children with cancer or for those who have normal immune function.

Recommendations for Personnel ▶ The most important practice that personnel can follow in caring for any child is careful handwashing. Indeed, whether the child has normal immunity or abnormal immune function, the transmission of a variety of common infections, including respiratory viruses and gastrointestinal viruses (including hepatitis), could be reduced if careful handwashing is practiced. Furthermore, staff members should instruct children to wash their hands, particularly after toileting. Staff, of course, should always wash their hands between diaper changes or when assisting children with their toileting activities. When there is a known infectious hazard and staff must come in contact with soiled diapers, disposable gloves should be worn by the staff member and hands washed after glove removal. It must be underscored that wearing gloves is not a substitute for careful handwashing.

In urban areas where the risk for having a child with either HIV disease, tuberculosis, or hepatitis B is higher, staff should be informed about the potential infectious hazards as well as their routes of transmission. To that regard, staff must also be comfortable with the reality that the transmission of HIV virus by the kinds of contact that take place in a daycare or preschool setting is virtually impossible. Nonetheless, staff should exercise the principles of standard precautions when handling bloody secretions or a bleeding lesion. As noted above, spilled blood should be cleaned with a dilute solution of bleach and water.

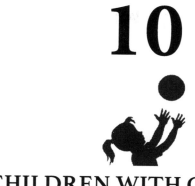

CHILDREN WITH CHRONIC LUNG DISEASE

Leigh B. Grossman

INFECTIOUS RISKS

Children with cystic fibrosis (CF), asthma, bronchopulmonary dysplasia (BPD), or other chronic pulmonary disease are not at increased risk of acquiring infection. However, they are at increased risk of developing severe and even life-threatening illness with organisms that ordinarily cause mild upper respiratory infection, bronchitis, flu, and pneumonia in the healthy child.

COMMON INFECTIONS

Unless there are other aspects to their disease that make them immunocompromised (e.g., corticosteroid therapy, asplenia, acquired immunodeficiency syndrome, transplantation, or cancer therapy), the causes of infection in children with chronic lung disease do not differ from those of their family or other healthy children in the daycare center or preschool.

INFECTION CONTROL

Special Infection Control Needs ▶ Preventing infection is the hallmark of effective infection control for this group of children.

Vaccine prevention of preventable causes of infection is imperative, and this specifically includes pneumococcal vaccine, *Haemophilus influenzae* type b vaccine, and yearly immunization with influenza vaccine. Respiratory syncytial virus (RSV) infection is common in the daycare setting and is a very high-risk pathogen for the infant with chronic lung disease. Preventive immunotherapies should be discussed with the child's physician. If possible, the infant with chronic lung disease should have a limited number of caretakers who thus minimize the child's exposure to a large number of different germs. Consideration should be given to avoiding group daycare during the times when many children at the center or school have upper respiratory illness (e.g., influenza season). In the case of the child with CF who is infected with a specific bacterium called *Burkholderia cepacia*, other children with CF are at risk of becoming infected with this pathogen and thus should not be in contact with the infected child.

Risks to Healthy Children ► There are no unusual infectious risks caused by children with chronic pulmonary disease. These children may carry unusual pulmonary and upper respiratory bacteria, but these organisms are not causative of disease in healthy children.

Exclusion from Daycare or Preschool Attendance ► Children with pulmonary disease who have worsening of their pulmonary symptoms (turning blue, grunting, altered breathing, increase in cough, vomiting) should be evaluated promptly by their physician. They should not be monitored in the daycare or preschool setting.

Exclusion for infectious diseases should be guided by the recommendations for all children (note Chapter 6 and the specific infection in Part V), realizing that children with chronic pulmonary problems may have a prolonged and more serious course.

Recommendations for Personnel ► All personnel should receive annual influenza immunization to minimize their likelihood of developing infection and then spreading infection to high-risk infants and children. Personnel should be extremely cautious in caring for the child with chronic lung disease to ensure that mild infection in themselves or other attendees is not spread to these children. This is best achieved through careful handwashing, particularly after caring for children with other viral respiratory illnesses.

Parental Advice ▸ Parents of healthy children should be told that children with chronic lung disease pose no unusual infectious risks to healthy children.

Parents of a child with chronic pulmonary disease should monitor their child for signs and symptoms of increased respiratory distress, particularly during seasons of increased viral respiratory illnesses. Parents should consider alternate daycare settings where their child avoids group daycare during times when many children at the center have upper respiratory illnesses. Parents should ideally have their child with chronic pulmonary disease cared for by a limited number of caregivers who receive annual influenza vaccination.

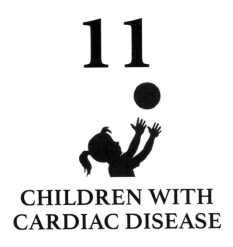

CHILDREN WITH CARDIAC DISEASE

Karen S. Rheuban

INFECTIOUS RISKS

Children with congenital heart disease often do not tolerate significant respiratory infections. The mortality rate of patients with respiratory syncytial virus (RSV) and underlying congenital heart disease is high. Because pulmonary function is already reduced in the baseline state, patients with abnormal intracardiac flow and resulting "wet lungs" or pulmonary edema do not tolerate acute pneumonitis and other lower respiratory tract infections.

COMMON INFECTIONS

The infections of children with heart disease do not differ from those of their surrounding family members. The exceptions include the child who also has asplenia (no spleen or no splenic function) or is immunosuppressed following heart transplantation, in which case overwhelming bacterial infection (bacteremia and meningitis) may occur.

INFECTION CONTROL

Special Infection Control Needs ▶ Prevention of infection is key to the management of children with heart disease in the daycare setting. Immunization against common infectious agents such as influenza, *Haemophilus influenzae* type b, and pneumococcus will prevent a significant number of infections known to worsen the course of children with congestive heart failure and will help prevent overwhelming infection in children with no spleen or no splenic function. Respiratory syncytial virus infection is common in the daycare setting and is a very high-risk pathogen for the infant with congenital and, particularly, cyanotic congenital cardiac disease. Preventive immunotherapies should be discussed with the child's physician. Immunosuppressed patients such as those following heart transplanation are at particular risk when exposed to the chickenpox virus and should not be immunized with live virus vaccines. Children with a history of rheumatic fever with cardiac involvement are at risk of recurrence of rheumatic fever when reinfected with group A beta hemolytic streptococci and should, therefore, receive prophylaxis in the form of oral or intramuscular penicillin. Patients with congenital and acquired heart disease should receive antibiotic prophylaxis against bacterial endocarditis for dental and other invasive procedures, most of which would not be relevant to the daycare setting unless in an emergency.

Careful handwashing should be practiced at all times, but emphasized when a viral illness is prevalent in the daycare center or the preschool. If at all possible, the infant with significant heart disease should receive care from a limited number of caretakers during outbreaks of upper and lower respiratory viral infections.

12

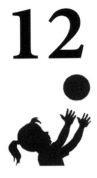

CHILDREN WITH DISABILITIES

Susan M. Anderson

Children with physical disabilities from:

- cerebral palsy
- genetic syndromes
- acquired brain or spinal cord injury
- myelomeningocele
- infections
- trauma
- burns

Children with cognitive impairment from:

- genetic syndromes
- acquired brain injury
- infections
- autism

Children with sensory impairments from:

- blindness
- deafness

– all may be provided care within a daycare or preschool setting.

There are more children with cognitive disabilities than children with motor disabilities, although at younger ages the cognitive disabilities may not yet be evident.

INFECTIOUS RISKS

Children with disabilities are at increased risk of infection for several reasons. Children with severe motor impairment may be at increased risk secondary to both general immobility and ineffective neurologic control of critical musculature. A child who is both immobile and has impaired control of the muscles of the throat and chest may be less able to cough and clear respiratory secretions and thus be at risk of aspiration and pulmonary infection. Children with severe immobility may be more prone to ear infections, particularly if their head is frequently in a dependent position and they are not able to clear oral secretions. Children with spinal cord injuries or myelomeningocele, because they have bladder dysfunction, are at increased risk of bladder colonization and urinary tract infection.

Children with disabilities may also have reduced ability to manifest or express their symptoms. Pain is a frequent sign that accompanies infection. Some children may be unable to communicate symptoms effectively because of oral motor dysfunction or language delay. In addition, there may be the loss of physical ability to demonstrate specific symptoms. Children with abnormal bladder function, despite having an increased incidence of urinary tract infections, often do not have the classic symptoms of urinary tract infection, such as frequency, urgency, and pain on urination due to their lack of sensation. Children with specific brain injury or cervical level spinal cord injury may have ineffective temperature control and may not demonstrate fever. Children who are on the autism spectrum often do not demonstrate or report pain due to difficulties with sensory integration. In addition, children with disabilities may be less likely to receive well childcare or be completely immunized because health care providers may be so invested in the child's special needs that routine health care is inadvertently overlooked.

COMMON INFECTIONS

There is no increase in the number of upper respiratory infections in children with disabilities. However, the occurrence of an upper respiratory infection in a child with oral motor dysfunction may compound the difficulty the child already has in handling their oral secretions. There is an increased incidence of ear infections in children with cleft palate, secondary to their palatal abnormality. There is also an increased incidence of ear infections in children with Down syndrome, secondary to their shortened and relatively horizontal eustachian tubes. There is an increased incidence of ear infections in children with oral motor dysfunction related to their inability to handle oral secretions.

As for lower respiratory infections, there is an increased incidence of aspiration pneumonia in some children with motor disabilities secondary to both oral motor dysfunction and the increased incidence of gastroesophageal reflux (GERD). Many of these children have a disordered swallow secondary to oral motor dysfunction and are unable to protect their airway. Children with impaired function of respiratory musculature such as those with neuromuscular disease or cervical-thoracic spinal cord injury are more likely to develop pneumonia and debilitating lung disease if they acquire any respiratory tract infection. Therefore, yearly vaccination for influenza and routine immunization for *Haemophilus influenzae* type b, pertussis, and pneumococcus are important preventive measures in this high-risk population.

Children with disabilities are just as likely as other children to have viral gastroenteritis, but they are more likely than other children to have complications such as dehydration secondary to their inability to take enough replacement fluids by mouth.

In children with abnormal bladder function (commonly seen with myelomeningocele or spinal cord injury), there is an increased incidence of significant bacterial colonization of the urinary tract. Due to their lack of normal sensation, children with abnormal bladder function often do not complain of pain on urination, increased urination or urgency but may present with the history of a change in color or odor of their urine or symptoms of fever, vomiting, or abdominal pain. There is an increased incidence of urinary tract infection with significant immobility, as might be seen with severe cerebral palsy or prolonged casting (e.g., spica cast).

Children with disabilities are just as likely as other children to have childhood meningitis. Children with central nervous system shunts for hydrocephalus have an increased incidence of bacterial meningitis or ventriculitis (often with skin flora or unusual organisms) secondary to the presence of the shunt.

Skin infections may be more common in certain subgroups of disabled children. Decubitus ulcers (bed sores) may develop in children with spinal cord injury or myelomeningocele secondary to their loss of sensation. Cellulitis and impetigo may be more likely in children who are cognitively impaired or have severe autism because of repeated self-stimulatory or self-injurious behavior.

INFECTION CONTROL

Special Infection Control Needs ▶ For children who have disabilities, the most important infection control procedures are those that apply to any child, such as good handwashing. In addition, there should be appropriate education of all day-care staff regarding those signs and symptoms of infection to which any particular child in their care is prone. For example, those who are caring for a child with a myelomeningocele deformity should be aware of the signs and symptoms of urinary tract infection and meningitis/ventriculitis as children with myelomeningocele commonly develop these infections. Additionally those providing care for a child with myelomeningocele should be expected to provide vigilant skin care, particularly in the diaper region, as these children are also more likely to develop cellulitis, diaper rash, and decubitis ulcers without demonstrating any signs of pain.

Children with HIV infection may have cognitive or motor disabilities, which are often progressive in nature. The child with HIV infection, because he or she is immunocompromised, may have some risk of acquiring infection from other children in the daycare setting.

There is no risk to other children or daycare staff who have casual contact with the child with HIV infection. Should a child with HIV have a playground injury which includes bleeding, standard precautions should be utilized in cleaning the area and caring for the child.

Children with congenital cytomegalovirus (CMV) may have motor, cognitive, or sensory disabilities. Children with congenital CMV may excrete virus for a prolonged time following their birth. However, the majority of children in daycare who excrete CMV are those who acquire the infection postnatally. For this reason, children with congenital CMV should not be singled out for isolation or exclusion. No special measures are indicated except good handwashing.

Children with congenital rubella most commonly have visual, hearing, or cognitive impairments. Children with congenital rubella are able to transmit the rubella virus to susceptible contacts until they are 12 months of age or until they have documented negative nasopharyngeal and urine cultures after 3 months of age. Although other infants in a daycare environment may have acquired passive immunity from their mother, older infants, unimmunized children, children of unimmunized mothers, and daycare staff may be included among susceptible contacts. Because 10 to 15 percent of the adult population is rubella-susceptible, all susceptible daycare providers and preschool staff should be immunized.

Children with congenital herpes may have recurrent skin or mouth lesions but do not need to be excluded from childcare or preschool settings. Herpetic lesions should be covered with a dressing. Because oral herpes is extremely common and those who are infected may shed the virus between bouts of their fever blisters, there is no need to exclude these children.

Risks to Healthy Children ▶ Healthy children are only at risk of acquiring infection from children with disabilities in those special circumstances that have been described in which the disability is of an infectious etiology. Be careful, however, not to assume that all children whose disability was originally caused by infection places other children at risk. For example, a child who has cerebral palsy resulting from an episode of

H. influenzae meningitis in infancy is no longer infected and thus is not an increased infectious risk to healthy children.

Exclusion from Daycare or Preschool Attendance ▸ A child should be excluded from a daycare center or preschool if the treatment of the disease is not consistent with the normal function of the daycare setting. For example, a child with a kidney infection may require hospitalization and intravenous antibiotic therapy. If a daycare center or preschool is unable to provide the environment and resources to maintain the intravenous catheter, then this child should be excluded from the childcare setting until this special medical treatment is no longer required.

A child should be excluded from a daycare or preschool setting if that individual child's health is at significant risk secondary to his or her presence in that setting. For example, a child with acquired immunodeficiency syndrome (AIDS) who is immunocompromised may himself be at risk by being in close proximity to other children. However the child who has an HIV infection and is not immunocompromised may be able to attend preschool without any risk to his health.

A child should be excluded from attendance at a daycare if the child's presence in the center places other children at risk for infection. A child who is both a chronic biter and has hepatitis B may infect other children through biting. Children who are actively shedding rubella virus in an environment where there are many susceptible individuals may infect others through secretion and aerosol exposure; however, susceptible individuals may protect themselves through immunization.

Recommendations for Personnel ▸ Routine health care maintenance is of primary importance in a daycare center or preschool that provides care to disabled children. Personnel should understand all pertinent diagnoses and the risks for each child in language understandable to all caretakers.

Childcare providers should have an understanding of each individual child's disability and associated complications such that the signs and symptoms of infection in the child will be recognized. Emergency phone numbers should be maintained for primary physicians and other subspecialty physicians. As with all children, the immunization status of each child with disabilities should be determined. In certain situations (such as progressive or degenerative neurologic disease), the primary physician may have recommended that certain immunizations not be given.

The most important factor in the prevention of infection in children both with and without disabilities is good hand-washing.

Parental Advice ▶ All parents should understand that children with disabilities are no more likely to transmit infections to other children than are children without disabilities; a child cannot catch a disability from another child. Parents should be aware of the health, safety, and illness policies of the center and should make certain that their own child and all children in the center are fully immunized.

13

CHILDREN WITH CHRONIC SKIN DISEASE

(Eczema)

Patricia Treadwell

INFECTIOUS RISKS

Eczema (atopic dermatitis) is a chronic skin condition which affects 15 to 20 precent of children in the United States. With this incidence, it is likely that eczema will be noted with some frequency in a daycare center or preschool. Recently, a specific genetic mutation has been described which is associated with abnormalities of the skin barrier which predispose children with eczema to colonization and infection.

COMMON INFECTIONS

The majority of children with eczema have *Staphylococcus aureus* on their skin (colonized) which is either methicillin sensitive (MSSA) or less often, methicillin resistant (MRSA). Intermittently, these organisms may cause disease. Children with eczema also may become secondarily infected with viruses including herpes simplex (eczema herpeticum) and vaccinia (smallpox vaccine virus transmitted to the children of vaccinated military personnel).

INFECTION CONTROL

Special Infection Control Needs ▸ When the child with chronic skin disease is infected with certain organisms, special precautions may be necessary to prevent the spread to other children. Treatment of the eczema should continue, since the anti-inflammatory treatment in itself will reduce the number of organisms. Conversely, when children without eczema or other personnel in the center have certain skin infections, especially fever blisters (herpes simplex cold sores), and impetigo, the child with eczema should be protected from close contact with these individuals. Medical treatment is available for these infections, but in specific instances, such as with eczema herpeticum, the child with chronic skin disease may have to be excluded from the center temporarily. The primary physician would be the best person to make this decision.

Risks to Healthy Children ▸ If the child with eczema has an infection in a non-covered area, there is a potential risk of spread. Areas of infections should be kept covered, if possible, and all contact with wound drainage should be avoided.

Exclusion from Daycare or Preschool Attendance ▸ Children are excluded from the center or preschool only when they are considered to be contagious. This is usually the case when they have infection with herpes simplex or vaccinia. In addition, if the child has a serious bacterial infection with *S. aureus* and the child is not being adequately treated, temporary removal from the daycare or preschool setting would be appropriate. In general, children with eczema should be treated like all other children at the center.

Recommendations for Personnel ▸ The personnel need to be aware of the special needs of the child with eczema, which often include needs not necessarily related to infection (dietary, exercise, clothing) but which may exacerbate the skin condition, allowing for an increased risk of infection. In addition, the personnel need to be aware of what types of infections these children may develop.

Parental Advice ▸ Parents of well children should be advised that eczema in and of itself is not contagious. If a child with eczema requires therapy for an infection, like any other child at the center or school, the child should receive treatment and return only when there is no longer an infection risk to the other children.

14

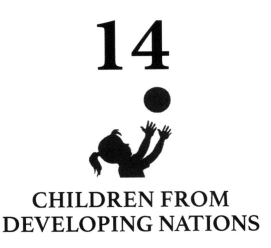

CHILDREN FROM DEVELOPING NATIONS

Leigh B. Grossman

INFECTIOUS RISKS

Children from developing nations often come from regions where sanitation is poor and diseases are transmitted by food and drink contaminated by disease causing organisms. Overcrowding and malnutrition may lead to an increased incidence of other diseases, such as tuberculosis. In many developing countries, low immunization rates result in an increased incidence of polio, measles, meningococcal infection, and diphtheria.

Because these diseases are highly contagious during their acute stages and may be imported by visitors and immigrants, it is important to protect children in daycare settings by ensuring that all children receive all of the routinely recommended vaccines.

There are several organisms that a previously infected child can continue to carry and excrete for some time after the acute symptoms have resolved. In a daycare center or preschool, it is these organisms, excreted for relatively long periods, that pose the most risk of child-to-child transmission.

COMMON INFECTIONS

Pathogenic organisms potentially carried for prolonged periods by children from developing nations are:

Bacteria

- Salmonella
- Shigella
- *Campylobacter jejuni*
- *Mycobacterium tuberculosis*

Viruses

- Hepatitis A virus
- Hepatitis B virus
- Hepatitis C virus
- Cytomegalovirus
- Human immunodeficiency virus
- Poliovirus
- Enteroviruses

Parasites

- Protozoa
- Cryptosporidium
- *Cyclospora cayetanensis*
- *Giardia lamblia*
- *Entamoeba histolytica*
- *Dientamoeba fragilis*
- Plasmodia (malaria)

Worms

- *Hymenolepis nana* (dwarf tapeworm)
- *Trichuris trichiura*
- Hookworm
- *Ascaris lumbricoides*
- *Strongyloides stercoralis*
- Schistosoma
- *Taenia solium* (cysticercosis agent)

Many of the organisms listed above are not transmissible directly from one child to another. The reason for the lack of transmissibility varies with the organism but it may be because the life cycle requires an intermediate animal host, the eggs must mature in the soil before they are contagious, or the organism must be transferred very directly through sexual activity or infected blood or needles.

Therefore, common tropical organisms that are readily transmissible in a daycare center or preschool are:

Bacteria
- Salmonella
- Shigella
- *Campylobacter jejuni*
- *Mycobacterium tuberculosis*

Viruses
- Cytomegalovirus
- Hepatitis A
- Enteroviruses
- Poliovirus

Parasites
- Protozoa
- Cryptosporidium
- Cyclospora
- *Giardia lamblia*
- *Entamoeba histolytica*

Worms
- *Hymenolepis nana* (dwarf tapeworm)
- *Taenia solium* (cysticercosis)

INFECTION CONTROL

Special Infection Control Needs ▶ The majority of the organisms of concern are transmissible by the fecal–oral route (except for cytomegalovirus and *M. tuberculosis*). Therefore, infection control should focus on good personal hygiene, good handwashing, the preparation of food by staff who do not care for children in diapers, separate food preparation and diapering facilities, and the exclusion of children with diarrhea that is not manageable and/or is associated with fever. These measures are not special and are recommended for every daycare center or preschool, regardless of whether or not it is attended by children from developing nations.

Children with tuberculosis are not contagious unless they are obviously ill with symptoms such as chronic cough and weight loss. A chronically ill child from a developing country should therefore be evaluated by a physician before the child enters the daycare center or school.

Risks to Healthy Children ▶ Healthy children are at theoretical risk of infection from the shorter list of gastrointestinal pathogens listed above. Practically speaking, the organisms most commonly transmitted are salmonella, shigella, cryptosporidium, *Giardia lamblia*, and hepatitis A. The risk of infection can be reduced by the routine use of good personal hygiene as discussed above.

Exclusion from Daycare or Preschool Attendance ▶ Children from developing nations should be excluded from daycare attendance when they have an unexplained chronic illness or when they have acute diarrhea. A child who repeatedly bites should be excluded until it is certain that he or she is not carrying the hepatitis B virus or the human immunodeficiency virus.

Recommendations for Personnel ▶ Daycare and preschool personnel should understand that there is little likelihood that a child from a developing country will pass along a dangerous disease to other children. Immunization for vaccine preventable diseases, good personal hygiene, and the exclusion of children with diarrhea that is not manageable and/or is associated with fever should be routinely practiced to minimize the transmission of disease.

Any child who appears to be chronically unwell should be evaluated by a doctor who has been informed that the child may have a disease that is prevalent in the developing world and be investigated accordingly.

Because hepatitis A is a more serious disease in adults than in young children, all personnel should receive the hepatitis A vaccine. Personnel should also ensure that they are fully immunized against polio.

Parental Advice ► It is important for parents to understand that:

- Children get diarrhea in daycare regardless of whether there are children in attendance from developing nations.
- Parents should make certain that there is good personal hygiene practiced in the daycare center or preschool before enrolling their child.
- Foreign children in the daycare or preschool setting are at minimal risk of spreading serious disease to other children.
- Parents should ensure that their children have received all the routine and recommended immunizations.

PART V

SPECIFIC INFECTIONS

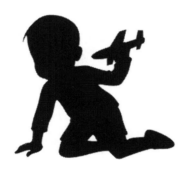

Robyn's Daycare Sends Home a Note

Robyn is a three year old with blue eyes and long blonde curls. She is sent home from daycare with her usual packet of art and notes. But today, one of the notes reports that the daycare center has a few children with lice.

Robyn lives with her mother and two school-aged brothers. Her mother immediately starts to itch! She wonders whether Robyn has the infection. Does she need to go to the doctor? Should she treat herself? Should she treat everyone at home? Should she fumigate the house? And, when can Robyn go back to daycare?

What should Robyn's mother do?

Part V of this book provides details about more than fifty infections – from Adenovirus to Yersinia – that parents of children in daycare and preschool may encounter. The expert authors explain how each infection is spread, what causes it, what signs and symptoms are clues toward a diagnosis, how the infection is treated, how long it lasts, and how long the child – and infected adults at the center – may need to stay home.

When Robyn's mother consults the chapter for Pediculosis (Lice), she discovers what to look for in Robyn and her brothers and herself, and what to do if she finds lice or nits in anyone's hair. She also is relieved to learn that, as soon as her daughter is treated, Robyn will be able to return to daycare.

HOW TO USE PART V

Part V allows you to look up each specific germ by name. Although we generally talk about symptoms such as sore throat or diarrhea, vomiting or headache, these same symptoms can suggest different infectious diseases such as flu, gastroenteritis, bronchitis, or colds and result from infection with many different causative germs.

We have chosen in this section to use the specific germ names since many of them may cause the same disease, but many of them have their own particular mode of spread, signs and symptoms, disease course, and infection control suggestions.

As you use this section, along with the Quick References in Parts I, II, and III, and the book index, you will have the tools to review how best to care for your child and his or her specific germ or disease.

15

ADENOVIRUS

Scott A. Halperin

SIGNS AND SYMPTOMS

Adenovirus is a common viral infection with diverse clinical signs and symptoms. Occasionally, these signs and symptoms are so distinct that a clinical diagnosis can be made with assurance. In most cases, however, adenovirus causes an illness indistinguishable from that caused by a variety of other pathogens.

Adenovirus most frequently causes infection of the respiratory and gastrointestinal tracts. It is an unusual cause of the common cold but a very common cause of upper respiratory infection with pharyngitis and fever. Adenovirus causes conjunctivitis (pinkeye), tonsillitis, laryngotracheitis (croup), bronchitis, bronchiolitis, and pneumonia. Adenovirus also is the cause of a characteristic syndrome called pharyngoconjunctival fever, which occurs in epidemics most commonly associated with contaminated swimming pool water. In addition to these infections of the upper respiratory tract, adenovirus is a major cause of childhood diarrhea. Upper respiratory symptoms also may occur in children with diarrhea caused by adenovirus infection.

CAUSE

Adenoviruses are nonenveloped, double-stranded DNA viruses. In humans, 51 different serotypes have been identified.

SPREAD AND CONTROL

Source of the Organism ► Adenovirus can be found in the respiratory secretions, conjunctiva, and stool of infected individuals.

High-Risk Populations ► Adenovirus infection occurs most often and is more severe in young infants and children. Outbreaks occur commonly in situations where close contact is common, including childcare centers, schools, and hospitals. Particularly severe epidemics occur in military recruit populations. Infections in immunocompromised patients are increasing, particularly in bone marrow and solid organ transplant recipients and patients with acquired immunodeficiency syndrome.

Mode of Spread ► Spread of adenovirus infection is by small-droplet aerosols. Infection is initiated when virus-containing particles come in contact with the nose, throat, or mucosa of the eye of susceptible individuals. Adenovirus is also spread by the fecal–oral route.

Incubation Period ► Two to 14 days.

DIAGNOSIS

In most situations, a definitive test for adenovirus infection is not made. Typically, a clinical syndrome such as conjunctivitis, croup, bronchiolitis, pneumonia, or gastroenteritis is diagnosed without a test done to identify the specific organism. A definitive diagnosis can be made through viral culture or through direct detection of the virus in clinical specimens using electron microscopy, immunofluorescence, enzyme-linked immunosorbent assay (ELISA), or polymerase chain reaction (PCR). Increasingly, real time PCR is being used for the rapid diagnosis of adenovirus infection. Specific diagnosis can also be accomplished by demonstration of an antibody rise to adenovirus in paired serum specimens.

TREATMENT

No specific therapy is available for the treatment of adenovirus infections. Most infections are not severe and do not require hospitalization; however, in the very young or immunocompromised patients, the infection may be severe and require hospitalization for supportive care. Cidofovir has had some success for treatment of adenovirus in the immunocompromised patient, but has significant renal toxicity.

INFECTIOUS PERIOD

Adenovirus can be isolated in respiratory secretions from 2 days prior to symptoms to 8 days after the onset of symptoms. Enteric adenoviruses have been identified in the stool from 3 days before diarrhea began to 5 days after diarrhea stopped, although excretion can occur for 2 to 3 months. Adenovirus can be cultured from the conjunctiva for 2 weeks after the onset of symptoms.

INFECTION CONTROL

Parental Advice ▸ Adenovirus infections are usually mild and self-limited. However, complications such as otitis media, dehydration, and pneumonia may occur, which would require a visit to the family physician.

Vaccine ▸ There is no commercially available adenovirus vaccine.

Exclusion from Daycare or Preschool Attendance ▸ No exclusion is required for respiratory infection due to adenovirus. The child's own condition should determine continued participation in childcare. Children with enteric adenovirus infection should be excluded from childcare until they are no longer having diarrhea. Adenoviral conjunctivitis often occurs in epidemics that are difficult to control; therefore, if an epidemic of keratoconjunctivitis is present, children should be excluded until purulent eye secretions have resolved.

Recommendations for Other Children ▸ Since exposure has already occurred before onset of symptoms, no specific steps need be taken once adenovirus infection has occurred. Each child should be monitored for any symptoms suggestive of more serious disease that may require a visit to the child's physician. The possibility of a more severe disease in immunocompromised children should be remembered.

Recommendations for Personnel ▸ There is no increased risk for adult caretakers due to adenovirus infection. Particular attention to handwashing and care with infected secretions, particularly stool, will prevent continued spread within the center.

16

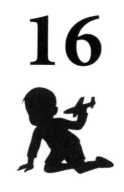

AMEBIASIS

Barbara A. Jantausch
William J. Rodriguez

SIGNS AND SYMPTOMS

Most amebic infections are asymptomatic. Some persons with chronic gastrointestinal infection with amebiasis may experience intermittent diarrhea, constipation, flatulence, vague abdominal complaints, cramps, and tiredness. Those persons in whom diarrhea develops usually have cramps.

Acute amebic dysentery occurs less frequently. The patient may have fever and dysentery (i.e., stools that are liquid and mixed with blood or mucus), abdominal pain, and chills. Headache, an urgent need to defecate, and leukocytosis may be present.

Ulcerative lesions in the gastrointestinal tract can, in less than 5 percent of patients, lead to the spread of the parasite to the liver, resulting in hepatic abscess. In approximately one-fourth of instances, enlargement of the liver with pain occurs. Jaundice is rare, but blood studies showing an increase in white blood cells and increased liver enzymes are common. A radiograph may show elevation of the right hemidiaphragm. Spread can occur to the lung, brain, and skin. On rare occasions, perforation of the large bowel, inflammation of the peritoneum, and death can occur.

CAUSE

Entamoeba histolytica is a protozoan parasite that has a global distribution. *E. histolytica* is now recognized as being two distinct species: *E. histolytica* and *E. dispar*. *E. histolytica* causes local and invasive disease, whereas *E. dispar* does not cause disease. The cyst is the infectious particle and is usually found in formed stool. After ingestion, cysts mature into active trophozoites that primarily remain in the liquid portion of the bowel contents.

SPREAD AND CONTROL

Source of the Organism ► Humans and primates are the reservoirs of *E. histolytica* and transmit the infection to animals including dogs, cats, and pigs. Food and water can be contaminated with amebic cysts, such that raw fruits and vegetables washed in contaminated water become additional sources of infection.

High-Risk Populations ► Distribution is worldwide but more prevalent in lower socioeconomic groups in developing countries. Travelers to these regions and children in daycare centers with infected children have potential for acquisition of disease.

Mode of Spread ► Fecal–oral transmission, person-to-person transmission, and ingestion of contaminated food and drink result in infection. Infection is transmitted by the ingestion of amebic cysts. Reservoirs of infection are those infected with no symptoms who may be shedding millions of cysts. Cysts are resistant to chlorination and can survive for several weeks in a moist environment.

Incubation Period ► The incubation period is usually 1 to 4 weeks but may range from just a few days to several months.

DIAGNOSIS

Intestinal Amebiasis ► The diagnosis is made on finding cysts or trophozoites on examination of fresh stool or bowel wall scrapings. Three stool specimens should be submitted 24 hours apart for evaluation, because cyst shedding may be intermittent. Cysts are more likely to be found in formed stool and trophozoites in fresh liquid stool. Preserved samples in PVA (polyvinyl alcohol) should be used if no fresh samples are available. *E. histolytica* and *E. dispar* have a similar appearance on stool examination. They may be differentiated by stool antigen detection assays, isoenzyme analysis, and polymerase chain reaction (PCR).

Acute Dysentery ► Mobile trophozoites with ingested red cells may be seen in dysenteric stools. Amebic ulcers may be seen on sigmoidoscopy. Serologic testing of blood, specifically the enzyme immunoassay (EIA) detects antibody to *E. histolytica* in the majority of patients with extraintestinal amebiasis, in patients with intestinal infection, and in 10 percent of patients shedding *E. histolytica* cysts. Positive tests may occur following appropriate therapy. Also available are enzyme-linked immunosorbent assay, immunofluorescence, and counterimmunoelectrophoresis. Serology is helpful in the dysenteric phase as well as in the extraintestinal phase.

Hepatic Abscess ► Antibody testing is very helpful (*E. histolytica*-specific IgG and IgA titers). In addition, imaging results provide useful diagnostic information. Elevation of the right hemidiaphragm may be seen in 50 percent of patients on chest radiograph. Ultrasound of the abdomen and computed tomography (CT scanning) can confirm the presence of a hepatic lesion.

TREATMENT

No treatment is necessary for *E. dispar* infection. Asymptomatic excretors with *E. histolytica* intraluminal infection should be treated with iodoquinol. Alternative therapy includes diloxanide furoate or paromomycin.

For intestinal amebiasis, liver abscess, or other invasive forms of disease caused by *E. histolytica*, metronidazole should be used in conjunction with iodoquinol or paromomycin. Corticosteroids and antimotility drugs should be avoided. Percutaneous or surgical drainage may be required in the case of a large liver abscess.

INFECTIOUS PERIOD

Individuals are infectious for as long as cysts are being shed in the stool. Untreated patients may excrete cysts for years.

INFECTION CONTROL

Parental Advice ▸ Parents should observe their children for gastrointestinal symptoms. Symptomatic children should be kept at home and be seen by their pediatrician, and their stool should be submitted for ova and parasite evaluation.

Vaccine ▸ None available.

Exclusion from Daycare or Preschool Attendance ▸ Infected children should be kept out of the daycare or preschool setting until they are treated and asymptomatic and their stools are free of oocysts. Stool enzyme immunoassays should be performed to determine if the parasite has been eradicated.

Recommendations for Other Children ▸ Children who develop gastrointestinal symptoms should be removed from the daycare or preschool setting, and their stools should be examined for *E. histolytica*.

Recommendations for Personnel ▸ Personnel should practice good handwashing, especially after using the toilet and handling diapers. Personnel who become symptomatic with gastrointestinal symptoms should remain at home and have their stool examined for oocysts. New children should not be admitted to the center during an outbreak.

17

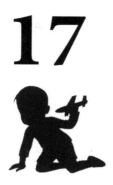

ANCYLOSTOMA DUODENALE

(Hookworm)

Jonathan P. Moorman

SIGNS AND SYMPTOMS

The initial manifestation may consist of itching and a bumpy (papular) or crusty (vesicular) rash at the site of larval penetration into the skin. While light infections often are asymptomatic, heavy infections may be associated with the development of abdominal pain, decreased appetite, diarrhea, and weight loss. Gastrointestinal symptoms appear to be more common in *Ancylostoma duodenale* hookworm infections than in infections caused by the other human hookworm, *Necator americanus*. The most significant consequence of hookworm infection is the development of iron-deficiency anemia due to blood loss in the gastrointestinal tract. The anemia may be associated with a pale complexion (pallor), listlessness, shortness of breath, palpitations, increase in heart size, and stunted growth. Other findings in hookworm infections may include low blood protein levels, an increase in the blood eosinophils, and blood in the stools.

CAUSE

A. duodenale is one of two species of hookworms that cause widespread human infection. Humans acquire hookworm infection by coming into contact with infective larvae present in contaminated soil. The larvae penetrate the skin or gut, pass into the bloodstream, and are carried to the lungs. They then penetrate the small airspaces in the lung, ascend the trachea, and are swallowed, ending up in the small intestine where they attach to the bowel wall and mature into adult worms. The adult worms produce thousands of eggs that are excreted in the stools, completing their development in soil. Under suitable conditions, the larvae will hatch and molt, becoming infective for humans.

SPREAD AND CONTROL

Source of the Organism ▶ Hookworms are found predominantly in tropical and subtropical zones, with *A. duodenale* predominating in southern Europe, northern Africa, northern Asia, and parts of South America. These areas provide appropriate environmental conditions for the development of hookworm eggs. The infective larvae are found in soil contaminated with human feces, and most infections result from direct contact with the soil, generally through bare feet. Rarely, food contaminated with *A. duodenale* larvae can serve as the source of the infection.

High-Risk Populations ▶ Individuals who have direct contact with fecally polluted soil in areas where *A. duodenale* is common will have a significant risk of acquiring hookworm infections. Children's propensity to play in dirt and to be barefoot increases their risk of infection. However, since effective transmission requires development of the larvae in soil, direct person-to-person spread of hookworm infection does not occur. Therefore, institutional or daycare settings should not increase a child's risk of infection.

Mode of Spread ▶ Transmission occurs through skin contact with soil containing infective larvae. In a few instances, food contaminated with larvae has been implicated in the transmission of *A. duodenale*.

Incubation Period ▶ The time interval between acquisition of *A. duodenale* and the appearance of eggs in the feces has been reported to range from 43 to 105 days. Considerable variability is also observed in the time between infection and the development of symptoms; individuals may develop gastrointestinal symptoms approximately 20 to 38 days following an acute hookworm infection.

DIAGNOSIS

The diagnosis is established by identifying characteristic hookworm eggs in the feces; *A. duodenale* eggs cannot be distinguished from those of *N. americanus*. Although direct microscopic examination of a fecal smear will generally be adequate for the detection of moderate and severe infections, concentration techniques may be required to demonstrate eggs in light infections. The larvae or adult worms are rarely seen in stool specimens.

TREATMENT

In countries where hookworms are endemic and reinfection is common, light infections often are not treated. In this country, hookworm infections are generally treated with either mebendazole, albendazole, or pyrantel pamoate. Although pyrantel pamoate and albendazole are recommended drugs, the U.S. Food and Drug Administration considers them investigational for this condition. These regimens appear to be well tolerated, but experience with them in children less than 2 years of age is limited; the decision to treat a child in this age group should be made on an individual basis after determining the potential risks and benefits of therapy. A repeat stool examination should be performed 1 to 2 weeks following therapy, and retreatment should be undertaken if hookworm infection persists.

In addition to the use of antihelmintic drugs, iron supplementation should be provided to individuals with significant anemia.

INFECTIOUS PERIOD

Without therapy, hookworm infections may persist for many years, although egg production tends to decrease over time.

INFECTION CONTROL

Parental Advice ▶ Parents should be told that the risk of person-to-person transmission is minimal. If the attendee appears to have acquired the hookworm infection locally, the need for sanitary disposal of feces and the potential for spread through contaminated soil should be reviewed with all of the parents.

Vaccine ▶ None is available although several candidates are currently being studied.

Exclusion from Daycare or Preschool Attendance ▶ Isolation is not indicated for children infected with hookworms. Since human-to-human transmission does not occur and the eggs passed in feces are not infectious, an infected child does not need to be kept out of any daycare or preschool setting.

Recommendations for Other Children ▶ Other children are not at risk of acquiring hookworm infection unless they are exposed to soil with infective larvae. Unlike the situation with many other enteric pathogens, children should not acquire the infection if they inadvertently ingest fecal material contaminated with hookworm eggs. Therefore, no additional precautions need to be undertaken for children in a center when one child is found to have hookworm infection.

Recommendations for Personnel ▶ Personnel should be instructed to continue techniques that decrease fecal–oral transmission of pathogens, including good handwashing and appropriate disposal of fecal material. In areas of the country where fecal contamination of the soil may be a problem, children in the daycare or preschool setting should not be allowed to wander barefoot or play in the soil.

18

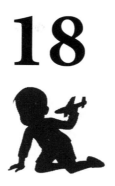

ASCARIS LUMBRICOIDES

(Roundworm)

Jonathan P. Moorman

SIGNS AND SYMPTOMS

The majority of Ascaris infections are asymptomatic, and symptomatic disease is proportional to the intensity of the infection. During the initial phases of infection with *Ascaris lumbricoides*, larvae migrate through the lungs. Infected individuals may be asymptomatic or have symptoms ranging from a mild transient cough to severe pneumonitis. In heavy infections, fever, eosinophilia, and pulmonary lesions may occur transiently with the pneumonitis. Once the larvae have passed into the small intestine and have matured into adult worms, ascariasis is generally asymptomatic. Spontaneous passage of the worms from the rectum, mouth, or nose may be the first indication of infection. Some individuals with ascariasis complain of vague abdominal discomfort, and a small number develop intestinal obstruction due to blockage by the adult worms. Movement of adult worms may occasionally be associated with intestinal perforation or blockage of the bile duct. Chronic ascariasis infection probably contributes to impaired nutrition and school performance.

CAUSE

A. lumbricoides is the largest intestinal roundworm parasit-izing humans. Infection is acquired through the ingestion of eggs containing infective larvae. After ingestion, the larvae hatch, penetrate the intestinal wall, and migrate via the blood or lymphatic system, passing through the liver and heart to the lungs. They then penetrate the alveolar walls, migrate through the upper respiratory tract, enter the esophagus, and pass into the small intestine, where they mature into adult worms. Female worms pass 200,000 eggs daily in the feces; these eggs, under appropriate soil conditions, can develop into infective larvae within 5 to 10 days. Unfertilized eggs or eggs that have not developed are not infectious.

SPREAD AND CONTROL

Source of the Organism ► Although *A. lumbricoides* has a worldwide distribution, it is most prevalent in areas with poor socioeconomic standards. Inadequate sanitation and the use of human feces as fertilizer contribute to the prevalence of asca-riasis by maintaining infective eggs in the soil. Transmission of the infection results from direct ingestion of soil, as in the case of some children, or indirectly through contaminated hands or food.

High-Risk Populations ► Preschool and young school-age children are at risk of acquiring ascariasis primarily because of their extended contact with soil and ingestion of soil either directly or indirectly through unwashed hands and food. This is reflected in the age distribution of ascariasis in areas with a high worm burden, where the prevalence increases sharply during the first 2 to 3 years of life.

Mode of Spread ► Transmission occurs through ingestion of *A. lumbricoides* eggs containing infective larvae. Since the eggs passed in human feces are not infectious until they have matured for several days to weeks in soil, person-to-person transmission does not occur.

Incubation Period ► The interval between acquisition of infection and the development of adult worms capable of passing eggs is approximately 8 to 12 weeks. Individuals who develop pulmonary symptoms do so approximately 5 to 14 days after infection, during which time the larvae are migrating through lung tissue.

DIAGNOSIS

During early stages of the infection, when the larvae have not matured into adult worms, the diagnosis may occasionally be established by finding larvae in sputum or stomach washings. Once adult worms are present, the diagnosis is readily established by finding A. *lumbricoides* eggs in fecal specimens. Occasionally, the diagnosis is made after the infected individual passes adult worms by mouth or rectum. A high eosinophil white blood cell count may be seen in pulmonary syndromes.

TREATMENT

Several relatively nontoxic drugs are now available for the treatment of ascariasis. Mebendazole, ivermectin, and albendazole are effective therapies but considered investigational for treatment of this parasite. None of these drugs have been used extensively in children less than 2 years old; therefore, the decision to treat a child of that age group should be made on an individual basis. In cases of intestinal obstruction due to ascariasis, piperazine citrate may be effective as this drug paralyzes adult worms, which may then be evacuated by normal intestinal motility.

INFECTIOUS PERIOD

In untreated individuals, A. *lumbricoides* adult worms may survive for 12 to 18 months. Individuals may asymptomatically shed eggs for years.

INFECTION CONTROL

Parental Advice ▶ The means of transmission, including the absence of person-to-person spread, for this roundworm is important. The need to prevent eating dirt (geophagia) and the requirements for good hygiene among all children is emphasized.

Vaccine ▶ None available.

Exclusion from Daycare or Preschool Attendance ▶ Children with ascariasis are not at risk of directly transmitting the infection to other children, and they therefore do not need to be kept out of the childcare setting.

Recommendations for Other Children ▶ Feces passed by a child with ascariasis is not directly infectious to other children. Therefore, other children in the center are at risk of acquiring ascariasis only if they ingest soil containing eggs that have developed to the infective larvae stage. To prevent potential transmission of a number of intestinal parasites, children should be kept from eating dirt, and good hygiene with handwashing should be emphasized.

Recommendations for Personnel ▶ Prevention of spread through the maintenance of good hygiene and appropriate disposal of all fecal material should be emphasized. Personnel should specifically be cautioned to avoid inadvertent contamination of hands, food, and utensils with soil potentially containing infective eggs.

19

CAMPYLOBACTER

Marian G. Michaels

SIGNS AND SYMPTOMS

Campylobacter jejuni is a major cause of gastrointestinal infection in both children and adults. The infection it causes presents in a similar fashion to many of the other gastrointestinal infections. Usually, infected individuals have rapid onset of diarrhea and abdominal discomfort of variable severity. Before the diarrhea, the child may have a fever followed by malaise and headache. Nausea often accompanies or just precedes the diarrhea. Blood in the stool is somewhat more common in Campylobacter diarrhea than in infections caused by shigella or salmonella, while vomiting appears to be a slightly less frequent finding.

Most often the disease usually lasts less than a week and goes away without any therapy. However, even when clinical symptoms have resolved, patients can continue to shed bacteria for 2 to 3 weeks, and even up to 7 weeks. This prolonged shedding is the reason why antibiotics are used for children in daycare or preschool.

Though complications are unusual, a protracted, relapsing course occasionally develops that can be confused with inflammatory bowel disease. Also, bloodstream infection, postinfectious arthritis, Reiter's syndrome, Guillain–Barré syndrome, carditis, megacolon, cholecystitis, and meningitis have been reported, albeit rarely.

CAUSE

Campylobacter is a bacterium that is a spiral-shaped rod that stains gram-negative. There are several different species, but the most common one to cause gastroenteritis is *C. jejuni*. In addition, *C. upsaliensis* has caused outbreaks of diarrhea in daycare centers in Brussels. *C. fetus* occasionally causes more overwhelming disease in premature infants and other immunocompromised hosts.

SPREAD AND CONTROL

C. jejuni has worldwide distribution. It is one of the most common causes of bacterial diarrhea in children, being more common than shigella and second only to salmonella as a cause of foodborne bacterial diarrhea in the United States. In temperate countries, infection occurs throughout the year, with peaks in the summer and early fall. The actual burden of of *C. jejuni* in a community is difficult to ascertain, as most people, even those with diarrhea, do not often have stool cultures. *C. jejuni* is not commonly found in the stool of asymptomatic people in the United States.

Source of the Organism ▶ Animal and bird species are common reservoirs for Campylobacter. Feces of migratory birds and domestic poultry have a high prevalence of Campylobacter species. Commercial chicken carcasses have often been found to be contaminated, as well as the carcasses of sheep, cattle, and swine. Campylobacter species have been found in surface water. In addition, *C. jejuni* can infect household pets and cause diarrhea in these animals, especially while they are young. Another source associated with outbreaks of *C. jejuni* enteritis is the consumption of unpasteurized milk or untreated water.

High-Risk Populations ▶ Daycare centers with children who are not toilet-trained are predisposed to transmitting Campylobacter infections in similar fashion to the transmission of other infectious diarrheal diseases. Children drinking unpasteurized milk or untreated water or those eating undercooked meat are at increased risk, as are those who have new puppies or kittens that have diarrheal illnesses. There is also an increased risk in people traveling to developing countries.

Mode of Spread ▶ Ingestion of, or contact with, contaminated food or water and fecal-oral spread are the primary modes of transmission. Children riding in the grocery shopping cart seat next to meat or poultry have also been implicated presumably due to handling of contaminated raw meat or poultry. Direct contact with infected animal or bird feces is also a method of spread. Maternal transmission of the bacteria to the newborn at the time of delivery has been reported.

Incubation Period ▶ Incubation is between 1 and 7 days, with most illness occurring 2 to 4 days after exposure, but this can be variable, depending on the number of bacteria ingested.

DIAGNOSIS

Diagnosis is made either by direct microscopic examination of fecal material using special stains or by isolation of the *C. jejuni* bacteria in stool culture. Stool specimens should be inoculated with minimal delay. If more than a 2-hour delay is anticipated, specimens should be stored using a special transport medium.

TREATMENT

The enteritis caused by *C. jejuni* is, in general, a self-limited disease often requiring only symptomatic treatment with oral rehydration fluids. The value of antibiotic treatment is controversial, as it does not appear to significantly alter the course of the disease. However, many studies demonstrate that despite continued symptoms, the shedding of *C. jejuni* is halted within 72 hours of administering antibiotics. Thus, in the daycare setting where children are not toilet-trained and transmission to other children is possible, it is prudent to treat with antibiotics.

Macrolides remain the drugs of choice for treatment of *C. jejuni*. Erythromycin remains the drug of choice with clarithromycin and azithromycin as alternative therapies. Systemic infections usually require hospitalization and administration of intravenous antibiotics.

INFECTIOUS PERIOD

Children are contagious for 2 to 3 days after appropriate antibiotics are begun. Those who have not been treated can continue to shed organisms in their stool for 5 to 7 weeks. Adults who have not had gastrointestinal symptoms have rarely, if ever, been implicated in the spread of *C. jejuni*.

INFECTION CONTROL

Parental Advice ▶ Parents should enforce good personal hygiene in their toilet-trained child. They can be reassured that their child does NOT require a stool culture unless he or she becomes symptomatic.

Vaccine ▶ None available.

Exclusion from Daycare or Preschool Attendance ▶ Two days after beginning antibiotics or until the child is asymptomatic, whichever is the shorter period of time.

Recommendations for Other Children ▶ Good hygiene.

Recommendations for Personnel ▶ Careful attention should be paid to handwashing after changing diapers and before food preparation. Toys and countertops should be cleaned more frequently, especially if used by children with diarrhea.

20

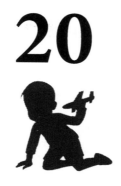

CANDIDA

(Thrush, Diaper Dermatitis)

Charles M. Ginsburg

SIGNS AND SYMPTOMS

The skin and the mucous membranes are the most common sites of involvement in infections caused by the various species of candida. In most instances, the infection is superficial and acute; however, in newborns and immunocompromised patients of all ages, the pathogen may be invasive and has the potential to cause disseminated or chronic disease.

Oral candidiasis (thrush), the most common infection caused by the candida species, is an acute inflammation of the tongue and oral mucous membranes that is manifested as white or grayish-white localized or diffuse patches or plaques on the mucous membranes. In severe disease, the lesions may extend to the angles of the mouth (perlèche), where fissuring and cracking may occur. The plaques are tightly adherent to the mucosa, and attempts to remove them generally produce bleeding and result in a tender erosion in the mucosa.

The diaper area and the intertriginous areas of the axillae, groin, and buttock crease are the most common sites for candidal invasion of the skin. Regardless of the area involved, the clinical appearance is similar; the affected skin is fiery red and, depending on the duration of infection, contains lesions that range from slightly raised red bumps to discrete eroded lesions with a red raised border.

Often, there are also discrete red or raised satellite lesions in areas that are separated from the primary site of involvement by normal skin. Candida also may infect the skin surrounding the nails of the hands and feet, particularly in infants and children who suck their thumbs or other digits. These lesions are similar to those that occur on other areas of the skin; however, the lesions are generally more swollen than those that occur elsewhere, and, often, there is drainage from the lesions as a result of secondary bacterial infection caused by strains of staphylococci.

CAUSE

Although there are multiple species of candida, one species, *Candida albicans*, is responsible for the majority of infections in normal hosts.

SPREAD AND CONTROL

Source of the Organism ▶ Candida species are ubiquitous in the environment, largely as the result of human-to-human transmission. The digestive tract, the vagina, and, less commonly, the skin are the principal reservoirs for the organism.

High-Risk Populations ▶ Newborns, immunocompromised patients, and those with chronic endocrine disorders such as diabetes mellitus are predisposed to infection with candida. In normal hosts, the organism has a proclivity to invade traumatized skin or mucous membranes or those areas of the skin that become macerated as a result of excess moisture.

Mode of Spread ▶ The mode of spread of candida is dependent on the age of the patient. Newborns generally acquire the organism from their mother's vagina during the birth process. By contrast, infants and older children acquire the organism from their mother's skin or hands or from unsterilized nipples, bottles, or pacifiers. Additionally, in situations where there are breaks in the mucosal or skin barrier, children may acquire the organism from other infected individuals.

Incubation Period ▶ The incubation period for candida infections is not known.

DIAGNOSIS

The presumptive diagnosis of most superficial candida infections can be made on clinical grounds. In instances where the diagnosis is unclear, a definitive diagnosis can be made by obtaining scrapings from the surface of the infected lesions for microscopic examination and for culture.

TREATMENT

Oral or superficial skin infection with candida may be treated with nystatin suspension, or if more widespread, with an oral antifungal agent. Additional important measures for treatment of skin disease consist of keeping the affected area dry and, possibly, administering a corticosteroid cream to patients already being treated with antifungal therapy who have severe, highly inflammatory cutaneous lesions. Caretakers of diapered infants should be reminded to change the diapers frequently, clean the skin with soap and water, and avoid occlusive pants, cornstarch, and baby powders.

INFECTIOUS PERIOD

Patients are infectious as long as active lesions are present.

INFECTION CONTROL

Parental Advice ▶ Since this agent is common and the severity of illness caused by this organism for normal hosts is small, it is unnecessary to inform parents of normal children that there are cases of candida infection at the center. Parents of children who are immunocompromised should be informed of cases of candida so that they can consult their child's physician to obtain recommendations about management of their child.

Vaccine ► None available.

Exclusion from Daycare or Preschool Attendance ► Since most children with candidiasis do not have systemic symptoms and their activities of daily living are not compromised, they may attend daycare or preschool without limitation.

Recommendations for Other Children ► If careful hygienic procedures are followed by the adult personnel in the center and the infected patient is on effective therapy, there is little risk to the other children in the center.

Recommendations for Personnel ► Normal hosts who work in the center are at little risk for acquisition of this germ, provided that careful handwashing techniques are utilized. This latter aspect is particularly important for personnel caring for children with oral or skin candidal infections. Immunosuppressed hosts who work in the center should avoid direct contact with infected children but may work with uninfected children, since the risk for aerosol transmission of the organism is minuscule.

21

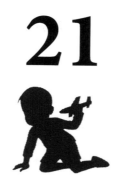

CHLAMYDIA

Margaret R. Hammerschlag

SIGNS AND SYMPTOMS

Chlamydia trachomatis: The major *C. trachomatis* infections in infants are conjunctivitis and pneumonia. The conjunctivitis may present in one or both eyes. The clinical presentation is extremely variable, ranging from mild conjunctival irritation and discharge to severe inflammation with chemosis, pseudo-membrane formation, and copious discharge. The conjunctival musoca may be very fragile and may bleed when stroked with a swab.

The clinical presentation of pneumonia due to *C. trachomatis* is very characteristic. The onset is gradual with runny nose and cough. The infants are usually afebrile. Physical examination reveals rapid breathing and wet lung sounds. Wheezing is distinctly uncommon. Chest radiographs demonstrate hyper-expansion and variable infiltrates. A very suggestive laboratory finding is a high blood eosinophil count.

Chlamydia pneumoniae: This Chlamydia species is a frequent cause of atypical pneumonia that is very similar in presentation to Mycoplasma pneumonia. Clinical manifestations include common cold symptoms, fever, cough, sore throat, and chest pain. *C. pneumoniae* also has been associated with otitis media and exacerbations of asthma.

CAUSE

C. trachomatis and *C. pneumoniae*: Bacteria that live inside cells.

SPREAD AND CONTROL

Source of the Organism ►

C. trachomatis: Among adolescents and adults, C. *trachomatis* is primarily a sexually transmitted disease. The adult genital tract is the major reservoir. In many adults, especially women, the infection is frequently asymptomatic and may persist for years if not treated. Newborn infants acquire the infection from their mother's birth canal during delivery.

C. pneumoniae: This organism is believed to be a primary human respiratory pathogen. The upper respiratory tract may be the primary reservoir. Preliminary clinical data suggest that *C. pneumoniae* may cause prolonged asymptomatic infection of the respiratory tract. Asymptomatic infection or carriage may occur in 2 to 5 percent of adults and children, but the role in the spread of infection is unknown.

High-Risk Populations ►

C. trachomatis: Since infection is acquired from an infected mother at the time of delivery, risk factors are those for infection in the mother: young age, early sexual activity, and multiple sexual partners. The institution of routine prenatal screening and treatment of pregnant women has resulted in a dramatic decrease in perinatal *C. trachomatis* infection among infants in the United States.

C. pneumoniae: Not known.

Mode of Spread ►

C. trachomatis: Transmission is from infected mother to infant during passage through an infected birth canal. If delivery is by cesarean section without rupture of membranes, transmission is unlikely to occur. There are no data supporting any form of mother-to-baby transmission after birth.

C. pneumoniae: Transmission is believed to be person-to-person by aerosol droplet or respiratory secretions. Outbreaks have been described in institutional settings, including military barracks and nursing homes. Spread within households has also been described.

Incubation Period ▶

C. trachomatis: Conjunctivitis – 5 to 14 days after birth; pneumonia – 14 days to 2 months of age.

C. pneumoniae: Not known. Some preliminary data suggest 3 to 4 days.

DIAGNOSIS

C. trachomatis: The diagnosis of conjunctivitis is made by isolation of the organism from a conjunctival culture or demonstration of chlamydial antigen by either direct fluorescent antibody test, enzyme immunoassay, or nucleic acid amplification test on conjunctival smears or secretions. Pneumonia is diagnosed by isolation of the organism from nasopharyngeal secretions obtained by swabbing or aspirating nasal secretions or by antigen detection or nucleic acid amplification methods. Serology is not useful.

C. pneumoniae: Culture of *C. pneumoniae* is performed in only a few laboratories. There are no commercially available U.S. Food and Drug Administration-approved serologic tests or nucleic acid amplification tests. Serology is of limited value in children.

TREATMENT

C. trachomatis: Conjunctivitis and pneumonia are treated with oral erythromycin (additional topical therapy is not necessary). Azithromycin appears to be as effective as erythromycin, although data are limited.

C. pneumoniae: Oral erythromycin is the preferred therapy. Alternatives include clarithromycin and azithromycin.

INFECTIOUS PERIOD

C. trachomatis: Not applicable, as child-to-child transmission does not appear to occur.

C. pneumoniae: Not known.

INFECTION CONTROL

Parental Advice ►

C. trachomatis: Parents should be reassured that C. trachomatis is not known to be transmitted child to child. Parents of infected children should be advised to seek treatment for themselves.

C. pneumoniae: Parents should be informed that this infection can progress to pneumonia. Children should be watched closely and brought to medical attention if symptomatic.

Vaccine ►

C. trachomatis: None available.

C. pneumoniae: None available.

Exclusion from Daycare or Preschool Attendance ►

C. trachomatis: It is not necessary to keep the child home, as child-to-child transmission appears to be very unlikely.

C. pneumoniae: The child should be on appropriate therapy and asymptomatic prior to returning to daycare or preschool.

Recommendations for Other Children ►

C. trachomatis: None.

C. pneumoniae: If infection is symptomatic, children should be taken to their physician.

Recommendations for Personnel ►

C. trachomatis: None.

C. pneumoniae: If infection is symptomatic, personnel should seek medical attention.

22

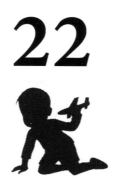

CORONAVIRUSES

(Common Cold)

Ronald B. Turner

SIGNS AND SYMPTOMS

The spectrum of clinical illness produced by coronavirus infection is not clearly defined. The major clinical syndrome caused by these viruses is the common cold. Colds produced by coronaviruses are similar to rhinovirus colds. Gastroenteritis has been suggested to be a symptom of coronavirus infection; however, this association has not been clearly established. Necrotizing enterocolitis has been reported in association with coronavirus infection of newborn infants.

CAUSE

The coronaviruses are RNA viruses. Four distinct human coronaviruses have been recognized; 229E, OC43, NL63, and HKU1. Severe Acute Respiratory Syndrome (SARS) is caused by an animal coronavirus that has produced infections in humans.

SPREAD AND CONTROL

Source of the Organism ▶ Infection with the human strains of coronavirus is limited to humans, and no animal or inanimate reservoir of infection has been identified. SARS originated from an animal source.

High-Risk Populations ► No populations have been identified that are at high risk for acquisition of infection. Newborn infants may be at increased risk of severe disease once infected. The factors that predispose to infection are not known.

Mode of Spread ► The limited data available suggest that coronaviruses may spread by small-particle aerosols. Further study is necessary to confirm this observation.

Incubation Period ► The incubation period for coronavirus colds is 48 to 72 hours.

DIAGNOSIS

Reliable methods are not available for the routine diagnosis of coronavirus infections.

TREATMENT

There is no specific therapy available for treatment of coronavirus infection.

INFECTIOUS PERIOD

The period of infectivity is not known.

INFECTION CONTROL

Parental Advice ► Coronavirus colds generally are mild upper respiratory illnesses, and no special precautions are necessary.

Vaccine ► None available.

Exclusion from Daycare or Preschool Attendance ► Exclusion from daycare or preschool settings is not necessary for children infected with human coronavirus.

Recommendations for Other Children ► No special precautions are indicated.

Recommendations for Personnel ► No special precautions are indicated.

23

COXSACKIEVIRUS A16

(Hand, Foot, and Mouth Syndrome)

Ziad M. Shehab

SIGNS AND SYMPTOMS

Hand, foot, and mouth syndrome is an illness characterized by the development of fever for 1 to 2 days followed by lesions in the mouth that are usually located on the buccal mucosa (inside of cheek), tongue, or gums. Shortly after the onset of the oral lesions, a rash develops that is characterized by small circular vesicular (crusty) lesions on the hands and/or the feet. The oral lesions are more commonly seen in children compared to adults. In addition, the buttocks are sometimes involved, but the rash there tends not to be vesicular. Resolution is usually complete within 1 week.

CAUSE

Hand, foot, and mouth syndrome is usually caused by the enterovirus, coxsackievirus A16. Other enteroviruses have also been associated with this syndrome, especially enterovirus 71.

SPREAD AND CONTROL

Source of the Organism ▶ Humans are the only natural host for enteroviruses.

High-Risk Populations ▶ Young children are particularly susceptible to this infection because of their lack of previous infection and immunity. Household members are also at increased risk.

Mode of Spread ▶ The virus is transmitted by the fecal–oral or oral–oral routes.

Incubation Period ▶ The incubation period is typically 4 to 6 days.

DIAGNOSIS

The infection is diagnosed based on the typical course and manifestations of the illness. It can be confirmed by testing throat swabs by culture or by specific PCR (polymerase chain reaction) tests.

TREATMENT

No specific therapy is available. Treatment is entirely symptomatic. Hospitalization is not required.

INFECTIOUS PERIOD

The infectivity of patients with hand, foot, and mouth syndrome is prolonged, spanning from before the onset of the oral lesions to weeks following resolution of the illness. Keep in mind that most infections are entirely asymptomatic.

INFECTION CONTROL

Parental Advice ▶ Reassure parents that this is a self-limited, mild, and, in most instances, asymptomatic infection with no serious sequelae.

Vaccine ▶ None available.

Exclusion from Daycare or Preschool Attendance ▶ Excretion of the virus in hand, foot, and mouth syndrome is prolonged, and most infections are asymptomatic. Therefore, removal of the child from daycare or preschool is not warranted and would have little to no impact on the spread of the infection.

Recommendations for Other Children ▶ Emphasize basic hygiene, specifically, handwashing.

Recommendations for Personnel ▶ Emphasize basic hygienic measures (e.g., handwashing) with all children and staff in the center.

24

CRYPTOSPORIDIA

Barbara A. Jantausch
William J. Rodriguez

SIGNS AND SYMPTOMS

Cryptosporidium causes severe diarrhea in patients with compromised immune function and is a self-limited disease in immunocompetent hosts. Cryptosporidium is recognized as a common gastrointestinal pathogen throughout the world, being more common in developing countries, and as a cause of diarrheal outbreaks in daycare centers and preschools in the United States.

Patients with normal immune function experience self-limited disease and have watery nonbloody stools, abdominal pain, and weight loss for approximately 10 to 14 days. Vomiting and cough can also occur. Fever can occur as well, particularly among young children. Rarely, patients may be asymptomatic carriers. Patients with altered immune function may have severe, protracted, or voluminous diarrhea resulting in dehydration and malnutrition and may experience disseminated infection.

CAUSE

Cryptosporidium, meaning "hidden spore" in Greek, is a protozoan parasite. The oocyst is the infective particle. Seventeen species of Cryptosporidium have been identified; *Cryptosporidium parvum* and *Cryptosporidium muris* have been associated with human infection.

SPREAD AND CONTROL

Source of the Organism ▸ The organism is found in the gastrointestinal tract of infected humans and animals, such as those in petting zoos, as well as reptiles, birds, and mammals, and in contaminated food and water and on contanimated objects. Community outbreaks have occurred as a result of contamination of municipal water supplies and swimming pools.

High-Risk Populations ▸ Persons at the highest risk for acquiring cryptosporidia are: immunocompromised persons; healthy homosexual men; travelers, especially to developing countries; animal handlers; household contacts of infected persons; hospitalized persons; children in daycare centers, preschools, and hospitals; and childcare personnel with exposure to infected children.

Mode of Spread ▸ Spread occurs through: fecal–oral transmission; person-to-person transmission; direct and indirect contact of infected feces; and contaminated food, water, and surfaces. The diaper changing area and mouthing of shared objects by infants and toddlers can be sources of the organism.

Incubation Period ▸ The incubation period is estimated to be between 2 and 14 days, with a median of 7 days.

DIAGNOSIS

The diagnosis is made by detection of Cryptosporidium oocysts in stool by using special staining techniques. An enzyme immunoassay test and polymerase chain reaction test are also commercially available. At least three stool specimens collected from different days should be submitted for examination. The organism can also be identified by light and electron microscopy of intestinal biopsy samples.

TREATMENT

The disease is self-limited in the healthy person. Nitazoxanide is approved to treat infection in adults and in children 12 months of age and older with diarrhea. Paromomycin alone or in combination with azithromycin have some reported success. Antiperistaltic (e.g., loperamide) agents have not been found to be beneficial and have been noted to worsen abdominal cramping and should not be used.

INFECTIOUS PERIOD

Oocysts may be shed in the stool of otherwise healthy patients for 2 to 5 weeks, although in most cases this stops within 2 weeks after resolution of symptoms. Immunocompromised patients usually shed oocysts forever.

INFECTION CONTROL

Parental Advice ▶ Parents should monitor their children for symptoms of diarrhea. Symptomatic children should be removed from the daycare or preschool setting, be seen by their pediatrician, and have three stool specimens submitted from different days for evaluation for oocysts.

Vaccine ▶ None available.

Exclusion from Daycare or Preschool Attendance ▶ Children should be kept out of the daycare or preschool setting until they are asymptomatic. They should refrain from recreational swimming and/or bathing for 2 weeks after symptoms resolve.

Recommendations for Other Children ▶ Children who develop diarrhea should have their stools evaluated for oocysts. Good handwashing, proper disposal of stools, and grouping of children with diarrheal symptoms should be practiced.

Recommendations for Personnel ▶ Personnel should practice good handwashing, especially after using the toilet and handling diapers. The organism is resistant to chlorine. Use of an ammonia solution to decontaminate the environment may inactivate cysts. Personnel who become symptomatic should remain at home and have their stools evaluated for oocysts. During an outbreak, no new enrollees should be accepted, and children with similar symptoms should be grouped to avoid infecting well children.

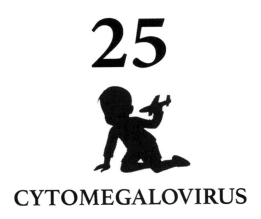

CYTOMEGALOVIRUS

Stuart P. Adler

SIGNS AND SYMPTOMS

The majority of children with infections due to cytomegalovirus (CMV) acquired after birth have no symptoms. Occasionally, and particularly in older children and adults, CMV will cause an infectious mononucleosis syndrome with sore throat, swollen lymph nodes in the neck, enlarged liver, rash, and atypical white cells in the blood. However, this is very rare, especially in young children in daycare or preschool.

CAUSE

CMV infects only humans. Only one major serotype exists.

SPREAD AND CONTROL

Source of the Organism ▶ The virus is acquired by transmission from human to human, and nearly all humans eventually become infected. Infections occur more frequently when there is crowding and intimate contact.

High-Risk Populations ▶ Everyone in the population eventually acquires an infection with CMV. In immunocompromised patients, infection can be severe and/or prolonged. Infection in susceptible pregnant women can result in fetal infection.

Mode of Spread ▸ The exact mode of spread of the virus is unknown, although we assume that intimate contact (e.g., diaper changing, kissing, feeding, bathing, and other activities that result in contact with infected urine or saliva) is important for spread. The virus will remain alive on surfaces and diapers for several hours.

Incubation Period ▸ The incubation period for this infection is approximately 1 month.

DIAGNOSIS

CMV infection is best diagnosed by obtaining a sample of urine for culture. Development of antibodies that are detectable in blood is also possible but requires a blood sample obtained before infection and one obtained after infection.

TREATMENT

Ganciclovir, valganciclovir, foscarnet, cidofovir, and fomivirsen may be considered for therapy in the immunocompromised patient with CMV infection. No therapy is recommended for infection in the normal child.

INFECTIOUS PERIOD

Most children who acquire CMV infections shed the virus for many months, with a range of 6 months to 2 years. Adults shed for a shorter period, probably less than 6 months.

INFECTION CONTROL

Parental Advice ▸ Pregnant women with a child younger than 2 years of age in group daycare or preschool should assume that their own child is shedding the virus and thus exercise careful hand-washing and scrupulous control of secretions and excretions. See the list below of suggested Practices for Susceptible Pregnant Women to Reduce Risk of CMV Infection. Routine testing of serum for IgG antibodies for pregnant mothers is not universally recommended although some women may want to assess their risk by determining if they are immune or susceptible.

Vaccine ▸ None available.

Exclusion from Daycare or Preschool Attendance ▸ Children excreting CMV should not be kept out of daycare.

Recommendations for Other Children ▸ No attempts should be made to prevent children from spreading CMV from child to child in the daycare center or preschool, as many children will naturally be infected with this virus.

Recommendations for Personnel ▸ Pregnant personnel should assume that all children are excreting the virus. If possible, at least 6 months before pregnancy, women should be tested to determine whether they have antibodies to CMV (immunity) and therefore are unlikely to give birth to a child affected by this virus. If a pregnant woman lacks immunity (tests seronegative) and is pregnant or attempting to become pregnant, it is suggested that she be assigned to work with children older than 2 years of age. If or when contact with children younger than 2 years of age is necessary, avoidance of contact with urine and saliva and avoidance of intimate contact (e.g., kissing, snuggling) is suggested. Use of standard precautions, including scrupulous handwashing technique and glove use, is required.

Practices for Susceptible Pregnant Women to Reduce Risk of CMV Infection ▸

- Assume children under age 3 years in your care have CMV in their urine and saliva.
- Thoroughly wash hands with soap and warm water after:
  ○ diaper changes and handling child's dirty laundry,
  ○ feeding or bathing child,
  ○ wiping child's runny nose or drool, and
  ○ handling child's toys, pacifiers, or toothbrushes.

- Do not:
  - ° share cups, plates, utensils, toothbrushes or food;
  - ° kiss child on or near the mouth;
  - ° share towels or washcloths with child; or
  - ° sleep in the same bed with child.

26

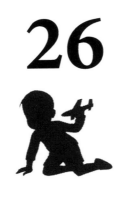

DIPHTHERIA

Leigh B. Grossman

SIGNS AND SYMPTOMS

Diphtheria may cause disease in the nose, throat, or large airways, or be limited to the skin. Diphtheria toxin can produce serious damage to the heart muscle, the nervous system, and the kidneys, resulting in life-threatening complications.

Tonsillopharyngeal diphtheria, or diphtheria of the throat, is the most common form of diphtheria and is manifested by a fever with a severe sore throat, generalized toxicity, and the presence of a yellowish, white filmy substance or exudate over the pharynx, tonsils, or uvula. This exudate becomes organized into a pseudomembrane and may spread to cover most of the throat.

In upper airway or laryngeal diphtheria, the exudate involves the larynx and produces life-threatening airway obstruction.

Nasal diphtheria is a mild form of the disease, often devoid of toxic manifestations, and is more likely to affect very young children.

Skin or mucous membrane diphtheria may be found in warm climates presenting as a shallow ulcer, often coated with a pseudomembrane.

CAUSE

The causative organism is *Corynebacterium diphtheriae*, a gram-positive bacterium.

SPREAD AND CONTROL

Source of the Organism ▶ Infection is limited to humans. Infected persons as well as carriers may spread the organisms by respiratory droplets. Carriers are usually contacts of infected individuals.

High-Risk Populations ▶ Crowding facilitates the spread of the organism. Unimmunized or partially immunized individuals are particularly susceptible to the disease, though immunization does not provide 100 percent protection.

Mode of Spread ▶ The organism is spread by intimate contact through nasal or oral secretions or contact with infected skin.

Incubation Period ▶ The incubation period for diphtheria is usually 2 to 6 days.

DIAGNOSIS

The diagnosis is based entirely on isolation of the organism from cultures obtained from infected sites. Isolation of the organism requires the use of special media both for transport and for growth.

TREATMENT

The cornerstone of therapy is the early administration of diphtheria antitoxin, which is only available from the Centers for Disease Control as an investigational drug. Antimicrobial therapy is important because it shortens the duration of communicability. Erythromycin is the preferred antimicrobial; penicillin is also effective.

Most infected children will require hospitalization for extensive support measures and monitoring of vital functions.

INFECTIOUS PERIOD

Untreated patients are usually infectious for 2 weeks but occasionally may harbor organisms for months. Antibiotic treatment usually eradicates organisms after 4 days. Elimination of the organism should be documented 24 hours after completion of treatment by 2 consecutive negative cultures from specimens taken 24 hours apart.

INFECTION CONTROL

Parental Advice ▶ All parents should be notified immediately of the occurrence of diphtheria in the center. Written recommendations should be distributed to all parents, and documented compliance should be required for return to the daycare center or preschool.

Vaccine ▶ All children attending daycare must be fully immunized against diphtheria. All previously immunized individuals who are exposed to a child with diphtheria should receive a booster of toxoid if their last dose of toxoid was 5 or more years before exposure.

Exclusion from Daycare or Preschool Attendance ▶ The infected child should be kept out of the daycare or preschool setting for at least 1 week after the start of antibiotic therapy. A negative culture should be documented before returning the child to the center.

Recommendations for Other Children ▶ A single case of diphtheria in a daycare or preschool setting would be unusual in a highly immunized population. An outbreak would be extremely unlikely and could create panic among parents and providers. Public health authorities should be notified immediately. It would be wise to have a meeting of all concerned to explain the issue and answer questions.

Children, providers, and the family of the first case must be cultured and placed under clinical surveillance for a week.

Those who have been immunized but have not had a booster during the preceding 5 years require a booster dose of diphtheria toxoid. Care must be taken to give only the adult type of toxoid to adults; either Td, or if not previously received, Tdap. Vaccine should be given to those who have not been previously immunized.

Additionally, all close contacts of the first case should receive antimicrobial prophylaxis with oral erythromycin or intramuscular benzathine penicillin G. Azithromycin has good in vitro activity against *C. diphtheriae*, but has not been evaluated in clinical infection or in carriers.

Recommendations for Personnel ▸ Personnel should be cultured and placed under clinical surveillance for 1 week. Those who have not been immunized should be immunized. Those who were immunized more than 5 years before exposure should receive a booster dose of diphtheria toxoid. Culture-positive individuals or very close contacts should receive 1 week of prophylactic antibiotic therapy with either oral erythromycin or injectable penicillin. Azithromycin has good in vitro activity against *C. diphtheriae* but has not been evaluated in clinical infection or in carriers.

27

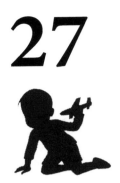

ENTEROBIUS VERMICULARIS

(Pinworm)

Jonathan P. Moorman

SIGNS AND SYMPTOMS

Most *Enterobius vermicularis* infections are asymptomatic. Anal itching is the most common symptom associated with enterobiasis and usually occurs at night, leading to restless sleep in many children. Symptoms may recur every 6 to 8 weeks, corresponding to the life cycle of the parasite. Much less often, vulvar itching may be associated with infection. In rare cases, migration of the adult worm from the perineum has been associated with vaginitis, and intra-abdominal inflammation. Although a number of other manifestations, such as loss of appetite, weight loss, abdominal pain, bedwetting, and teeth grinding, have been attributed to pinworm infection, no studies have indicated a causal relationship between those symptoms and *E. vermicularis* infections.

CAUSE

E. vermicularis, the human pinworm, is an intestinal worm. Humans acquire these worms by ingesting infective eggs. The larvae hatch in the intestines, developing into adult worms that live in the cecum and colon. Pregnant female worms migrate to the anus usually at night and deposit their eggs on the peri-anal and perineal skin. The females die after laying their eggs. Within a few hours, the deposited eggs are mature and capable of transmitting infection if they are ingested.

SPREAD AND CONTROL

Source of the Organism ▶ Pinworms, are the most common human worm infection, and infection occurs worldwide. The infective eggs, which are transmitted from person to person or indirectly through contaminated objects, appear to be relatively resistant to disinfectants and under optimal environ-mental conditions may remain alive for up to 13 days.

High-Risk Populations ▶ Due to their lack of hygiene, chil-dren are more likely to ingest E. vermicularis eggs and become infected than are adults. Therefore, pinworms tend to be prevalent in almost any setting where groups of children can be found. This includes large families, schools, daycare centers, and mental institutions. In these settings, the infection is often ubiquitous, with continuous transmission and reinfection of the children. Good personal hygiene can diminish the risk of enterobiasis, and if bathing and changes of undergarments are infrequent within a population, infection is even more likely to be a significant problem.

Mode of Spread ▶ Transmission occurs through ingestion of pinworm eggs with spread of the organisms via the patient's hands, especially the fingernails. Persons with enterobiasis may be reinfected if they scratch themselves and transfer eggs from their anal area to their mouth. Those in close contact with an infected individual may be exposed to contaminated objects. Transmission of E. vermicularis eggs can also occur through contact with soiled clothing or bed linens or through ingestion of eggs in house dust.

Incubation Period ▶ The time period between acquisition of infection and the deposition of eggs by the female worm has not been well established. Estimates range from 2 weeks to 2 months.

DIAGNOSIS

The diagnosis is established by detecting the eggs deposited in the perianal region. This is best done by applying transparent adhesive tape to the perianal region in the morning before a stool is passed or before a bath. After mounting the tape on a glass slide, it can be examined for the presence of pinworm eggs. The test may need to be repeated one or more times to rule out enterobiasis, with three tests detecting 90 percent of infestations. Less often, the characteristic eggs may be identified in a stool specimen, or the female worm may be observed in the perianal area at night. Eosinophilia or a specific white cell count, is not elevated in pinworm infection.

TREATMENT

Several effective and reasonably nontoxic drugs are available for the treatment of enterobiasis. Mebendazole, and pyrantel pamoate are the recommended therapies. Albendazole is also effective therapy but is considered investigational. It is recommended that treatment with these agents be given and then repeated in 2 weeks to eliminate any remaining adult worms. Most authorities recommend treating all individuals in the household of an infected child, while others recommend treating only those who are symptomatic or known to be infected. Limited data are available regarding the use of these therapies in children less than 2 years old; therefore, the risks and benefits of therapy should be carefully considered and a decision to treat a child in this age group should be made on an individual basis.

INFECTIOUS PERIOD

Individuals will have the potential of transmitting pinworms as long as they harbor adult male and female worms; although the female worm dies after laying her eggs, reinfection of the host is common, providing an ongoing source of adult worms.

INFECTION CONTROL

Parental Advice ▶ Parents should understand that enterobiasis is common and often unavoidable among children in any group setting. They should be educated regarding the mode of transmission, signs and symptoms, means of diagnosis, and therapeutic options. Lastly, they should be reassured that the diagnosis of pinworms in their child or in another attendee is not necessarily an indication of poor hygienic conditions.

Vaccine ▶ None available.

Exclusion from Daycare or Preschool Attendance ▶ Once the diagnosis of enterobiasis has been made, the child should be treated with one of the recommended regimens. After this one-dose therapy, the child does not need to be kept out of the daycare center or preschool.

Recommendations for Other Children ▶ Given the prevalence of enterobiasis, particularly within groups of children, it is highly likely that other children are also infected. Any children noted by parents or center personnel to have anal itching should be checked for *E. vermicularis* and treated appropriately if the infection is present.

Recommendations for Personnel ▶ Personnel should be made aware of the means of transmission and of the potential for them to be infected by the children. Good hygiene among the children and personnel with washing of hands, bedclothes, and toys should be emphasized. It should, however, also be understood that total prevention within a daycare center or preschool is very unlikely, if not impossible.

28

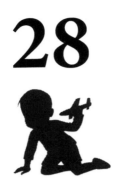

ENTEROVIRUSES

Ziad M. Shehab

SIGNS AND SYMPTOMS

Enteroviral infections are relatively widespread and include infections with polioviruses, coxsackieviruses, echoviruses, and enteroviruses. Infection with polioviruses results in an asymptomatic infection in 90 to 95 percent of cases. In addition, a minor illness may result. Occasionally, a viral meningitis (otherwise known as aseptic meningitis) can ensue. The most dramatic result of poliovirus infection is paralytic poliomyelitis.

The majority of infections with nonpolio enteroviruses are asymptomatic. The spectrum of illnesses caused by these viruses spans from asymptomatic to life-threatening. The occurrence of symptomatic illness is generally inversely related to age. Of the symptomatic infections, most are nonspecific and fairly minor febrile illnesses. Some specific rashes and oral lesions have been associated with them, such as herpangina, a febrile illness with oral lesions of the palate and tonsils, and hand, foot, and mouth syndrome.

Other diseases caused by these viruses include rashes, meningitis, respiratory diseases, gastroenteritis, conjunctivitis, and, rarely, inflammation of the heart, or paralytic disease.

CAUSE

Enteroviruses are RNA viruses that are ubiquitous. They are most prevalent during the summer and fall.

There are 65 serotypes of human enteroviruses. These include polioviruses, coxsackieviruses, echoviruses, and enteroviruses.

SPREAD AND CONTROL

Source of the Organism ► The only known reservoir of human enteroviruses is the human being.

High-Risk Populations ► Young children are especially susceptible to these infections because of lack of prior exposure. In immunocompromised children, enteroviruses can establish persistent infections.

Mode of Spread ► The virus is transmitted via the fecal–oral or the oral–oral route.

Incubation Period ► The incubation period is usually 7 to 14 days, although incubation periods of 2 to 35 days are not uncommon.

DIAGNOSIS

The diagnosis is established by virus isolation from a throat swab, stool specimen, and, occasionally, cerebrospinal fluid or blood, and only rarely by demonstration of a rise in antibody titer. Detection of virus by the polymerase chain reaction is now the preferred diagnostic modality.

TREATMENT

No specific therapy is available for enteroviral infection. The treatment is supportive care. In the more severe illnesses, such as meningoencephalitis, myocarditis, or poliomyelitis, hospitalization is often required. Bed rest and support for respiratory failure may be required in cases of poliomyelitis.

INFECTIOUS PERIOD

The infectivity of patients with enteroviral infections is prolonged, spanning from before the onset of the clinical illness to weeks following its resolution. Note that most infections are entirely asymptomatic.

INFECTION CONTROL

Parental Advice ► Emphasize basic handwashing hygiene. In the case of poliomyelitis, children whose immunizations are incomplete should receive polio vaccine, and inactivated polio vaccine should also be given to all household contacts.

Vaccine ► No vaccines are available for nonpolio enteroviruses. The inactivated poliovirus vaccine (IPV) is the only available polio vaccine in the United States.

Exclusion from Daycare or Preschool Attendance ► Excretion of the virus in nonpolio enteroviral infections is prolonged, and most infections are asymptomatic. Therefore, removal of the child from daycare is not warranted and would have little to no impact on the spread of the infection in this setting. Children with nonvaccine poliovirus infections should be kept out of daycare or preschool until shedding of poliovirus has resolved.

Recommendations for Other Children ► Emphasize basic hygiene regarding handwashing. In the care of poliomyelitis, children whose immunizations are incomplete should receive polio vaccine.

Recommendations for Personnel ► Emphasize basic hygiene measures (e.g., handwashing) with all children and staff in the daycare center. In the case of poliomyelitis, a booster dose of inactivated polio vaccine should be considered.

29

ESCHERICHIA COLI

(Diarrhea)

Barbara A. Jantausch
William J. Rodriguez

SIGNS AND SYMPTOMS

Disease caused by the various types of *Escherichia coli* is not very prevalent in the United States. Many of the diseases caused by *Escherichia coli* are more common in the developing countries where access to clean water and food is not reliable. However some strains of *E. coli* are seen in the United States and can be problematic in the daycare center or preschool. Most illnesses in young children present with crampy abdominal pain, watery diarrhea that may be bloody, some vomiting, and may or may not be associated with fever.

CAUSE

All *E. coli* are gram-negative bacteria. The five major types of *E. coli* disease and the usual diseases associated with these different types are:

Enterotoxigenic strains (ETEC): These produce either heat-labile, heat-stable, or both kinds of enterotoxins, causing disease by affecting the small bowel absorptive mechanism. This results in loss of electrolytes and water. Cramps, watery diarrhea, some vomiting, and very little if any fever are the hallmarks. Disease is self-limited and usually lasts 5 days. Enterotoxigenic strains are a common cause of traveler's diarrhea and diarrhea in infants in developing countries.

Enteropathogenic strains (EPEC): These *E. coli* strains are serotypeable but not enterotoxigenic or invasive. Those strains destroy the surface and digestive enzymes in the small intestine resulting in malabsorption. Although they usually cause self-limited disease in older children and adults, younger children and infants may have prolonged diarrhea lasting 2 weeks or longer. These latter patients may experience voluminous watery diarrhea without blood or mucus. These strains produce outbreaks of diarrhea in infants in the United States.

Enteroinvasive strains (EIEC): These strains cause a dysentery disease with a clinical picture comparable to that seen with shigella. These strains affect the colon and distal small bowel and produce enterotoxins which stimulate secretory diarrhea. Affected patients usually have fever, headache, and stool that may contain white blood cells and, less commonly, blood.

Shiga toxin producers (STEC): These strains, common in Argentina and South Africa, are represented in the United States in *E. coli* O157:H7. They produce Shiga toxin and create a syndrome characterized by severe abdominal cramps with a predominantly afebrile state accompanied by grossly bloody diarrhea and occasional chills. Hemolytic uremic syndrome (HUS) has been found to be associated with these strains. Gastrointestinal symptoms are usually self-limited and last about 5 days.

Entero-aggregative strains (EAEC): These strains have been postulated to be a cause of protracted (exceeding 14 days) watery diarrhea in the infant and young child and an infrequent cause of traveler's diarrhea in adults.

SPREAD AND CONTROL

Source of the Organism ▶ Infected persons and food or water contaminated with feces are the source of *E. coli* O157:H7, which is the most common of these *E. coli* strains in the United States. The organism can be transmitted by under-cooked ground beef and other products such as unpasteurized milk, contaminated apple cider, raw vegetables, and drinking water. Person-to-person transmission can occur during out-breaks. Hemolytic uremic syndrome, a syndrome associated with anemia and renal failure, can occur as a complication in 5 to 10 percent of children with *E. coli* O157:H7 infection; it can occur in higher proportions during outbreaks of *E. coli* O157:H7 infection.

High-Risk Populations ►

ETEC: Newborns, travelers.

EPEC: Newborns (uncommon), children in daycare centers.

EIEC: Those exposed to contaminated food.

STEC: Those exposed to infected persons, such as children in daycare centers, contaminated food, or water.

EAEC: Infants and young children.

Mode of Spread ► The organism is spread via fecal–oral trans-mission and person to person: caregiver to infant, patient to patient.

Incubation Period ► The incubation period is 10 hours to 6 days.

DIAGNOSIS

The diagnosis of these disease-causing strains of *E. coli* is made by bacterial culture, specific tests for the toxins, and tissue culture assays.

TREATMENT

Fluid and electrolyte supplementation is of paramount im-portance in treating any of these infections. Some types of *E. coli* are treated with antibiotics, but only with consideration to the possible complications associated with antibicrobial treatment in this population.

INFECTIOUS PERIOD

The infectious period occurs while the person is shedding the organism; it is generally considered to be while the person is symptomatic. The degree and extent of shedding may vary beyond that time.

INFECTION CONTROL

Parental Advice ▸ When *E. coli* is present at the center, parents should report even mild gastroenteritis symptoms in their child. Symptomatic children should be removed from daycare, seen by their pediatrician, and have their stool examined.

Vaccine ▸ None available.

Exclusion from Daycare or Preschool Attendance ▸ The child should be kept out of the daycare or preschool setting until he or she is asymptomatic and has negative stool cultures. In the case of *E. coli* O157:H7, the child should remain out of the daycare setting until the child is asymptomatic and at least two serial stool cultures are negative for *E. coli* O157:H7 or until 10 days after cessation of symptoms in the case of other *E. coli* organisms.

Recommendations for Other Children ▸ Close contacts of a symptomatic child with an invasive strain of *E. coli* may need to be cultured and, if their stool is positive, should be considered for treatment even if asymptomatic. In the event of an outbreak of *E. coli* O157:H7, the public health authorities should be notified immediately and the daycare center closed to new admissions.

Recommendations for Personnel ▸ Personnel should be grouped into those caring for sick and those caring for well children. Personnnel should practice good handwashing, and stay at home and be cultured if symptomatic. If initial contact measures are not successful, it may be necessary to close the center temporarily.

30

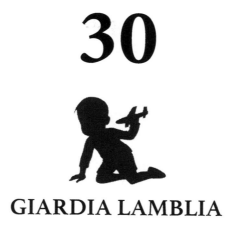

GIARDIA LAMBLIA

Theresa A. Schlager

SIGNS AND SYMPTOMS

Infants and children infected with *Giardia lamblia* can be either asymptomatic or symptomatic with either a brief episode of diarrhea or a chronic illness with multiple symptoms. An asymptomatic infection may be seen in as many as 50 percent of the infected children and increased rates of asymptomatic infection have been seen in daycare settings during outbreaks of diarrhea due to *G. lamblia*. Symptomatic infants and children with a brief illness will usually have diarrhea that is profuse and watery but unassociated with significant fever, toxicity, or dehydration, and that usually resolves without specific dietary alteration or drug therapy. Symptomatic patients who develop a chronic illness ordinarily have protracted, intermittent symptoms including watery diarrhea, abdominal cramps, a protuberant abdomen, wasted extremities, edema, significant weight loss, retarded growth, and anemia. Their stools contain an increased amount of fat but do not usually contain visible blood, pus, or mucus.

CAUSE

Giardia is a flagellated protozoan type of parasite. Only two species appear to infect humans. The protozoa exist in two forms: a trophozoite form that inhabits the lumen of the upper small intestine where it can cause symptoms, and a cyst form that inhabits the lower small intestine and the large intestine and, when excreted in stool, is infectious. When cysts are ingested by a susceptible host, trophozoites are released following the exposure of the cysts to the acidity of the stomach. The trophozoites can then inhabit the intestine, sometimes in very large numbers.

SPREAD AND CONTROL

Source of the Organism ▸ *G. lamblia* is distributed throughout the world and is the most common parasitic infection in the United States. Humans are the principal reservoir of infection, but dogs and beavers are other sources of infection. Feces or objects (toys, diaper-changing tables, eating utensils) soiled with feces or water or food contaminated with cysts are infectious by the oral route even if only small numbers of cysts are ingested. Most epidemics result from contaminated water. Prevention of waterborne outbreaks requires adequate filtration of municipal water obtained from surface water sources, because concentrations of chlorine used to disinfect drinking water are not effective against the cysts.

High-Risk Populations ▸ Infants and children in daycare centers or preschools are at high risk. In some areas, *G. lamblia* is the most common cause of diarrhea in daycare centers and preschools, both in outbreaks and in sporadic cases. The children most frequently infected are non-toilet-trained toddlers. Following daycare center or preschool outbreaks, 12 to 25 percent of family members of children (especially non-toilet–trained children) attending the center have become infected. There is increasing evidence that children in daycare centers are a common source for spread of *G. lamblia* to the surrounding community.

High risk children include:

- infants and children exposed to unprocessed water sources,
- patients with acquired immunodeficiency syndrome,
- patients with hypogammaglobulinemia,

- malnourished children,
- children who have had previous stomach surgery with removal of part of the stomach wall, and
- children with reduced gastric acidity.

Mode of Spread ► Infection is spread via the fecal–oral route. This requires the ingestion of cysts contained in feces, water, or food or on shared objects (toys, diaper-changing tables, eating utensils) contaminated with infested feces.

Incubation Period ► The incubation period is 1 to 4 weeks.

DIAGNOSIS

The traditional diagnosis of giardiasis has been by microscopic examination of the stool for trophozoites or cysts. Recently, rapid diagnostic tests that use antigen-detection methods have been widely employed. These tests are more sensitive and specific than microscopy in detection of giardia in stool samples. When giardia is suspected clinically but the organism is not found on repeated stool examination, examination of duodenal contents obtained by direct aspiration or using a commercially available string test may be diagnostic. Rarely, small bowel biopsy is required for diagnosis. Polymerase chain reaction (PCR) has been used to detect giardia in water systems and for rapid source tracking in epidemiologic studies.

TREATMENT

At present, only symptomatic infections are treated; the benefits and risks of treating asymptomatic patients have not been characterized. Several pharmaceutical agents available in the United States are effective therapy for giardiasis: tinidazole, metronidazole, albendazole, and nitazoxanide. Paromomycin, a nonabsorbable aminoglycoside, is less effective than other agents but is commonly used for treatment in pregnant women because of theoretical concerns regarding potential teratogenic effects with the other available agents.

If relapse occurs, therapy with any of the available agents can be repeated. Relapse is particularly common in immunocompromised patients who may require prolonged or combination therapy.

INFECTIOUS PERIOD

Patients are infectious for as long as they excrete cysts, and they may excrete cysts in their stools for prolonged periods (12 to 14 months). Excreted cysts may remain infectious for months if they remain in a moist environment.

INFECTION CONTROL

Parental Advice ► A daycare center or preschool should notify parents of children who have been in direct contact with a child who has diarrhea and from whom G. *lamblia* has been identified. Parents should contact their physician for advice if their child develops diarrhea or signs of chronic illness. Parents should encourage children to avoid swallowing recreational water and should avoid drinking untreated water during community outbreaks.

Vaccine ► A vaccine is not presently available.

Exclusion from Daycare or Preschool Attendance ► Children who have had symptomatic giardiasis who have completed a course of therapy should be allowed to return to the daycare or preschool setting when diarrhea is no longer present. The local health department should be notified.

Recommendations for Other Children ► Symptomatic, infected children should be treated. Routine testing is not recommended for children exposed to a child with G. *lamblia*. Washing of children's hands on arrival at the center, after a diaper change or use of the toilet, and before meals and snacks should be practiced consistently. Use of liquid soap in a dispenser along with disposable paper towels is recommended. Shared surfaces and toys should be disinfected on a daily basis with a freshly prepared solution of commercially available cleanser (detergents, disinfectant detergents, or chemical germicides).

Recommendations for Personnel ► Symptomatic, infected staff members should be treated. Without failure, staff members should practice careful handwashing (10 seconds with soap and warm running water) upon arrival at the center, after changing a child's diaper, after using the toilet or providing assistance to a child using the toilet, and before food handling. Disinfecting diaper-changing surfaces along with proper disposal of diapers is recommended.

31

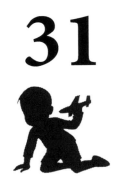

GONORRHEA

(Neisseria gonorrhoeae)

Michael F. Rein

SIGNS AND SYMPTOMS

In newborns, the most common presentation of gonorrhea is eye infection with drainage, which is often accompanied by asymptomatic infection of the throat. One may also see vaginitis, nasal discharge, penile discharge, or involvement of the sites where a fetal monitor was inserted. Among older prepubertal girls, vaginitis is the most common infection and presents as vaginal itching and discharge, both of which may be relatively mild. Infection may spread to the fallopian tubes, where it mimics lower abdominal pain from other causes. For prepubertal boys, as in adult men, the most common infection is acute urethritis, presenting as penile discharge and pain on urination. Oral or anal infections often remain asymptomatic. At any age, the organism rarely spreads to the joints, skin, meninges, or heart valves.

CAUSE

Neisseria gonorrhoeae is a gram-negative bacterium. It has become increasingly resistant to many antibiotics, and older treatments can no longer be used. The organism should always be cultured in pediatric cases.

SPREAD AND CONTROL

Source of the Organism ▶ *Neisseria gonorrhoeae* is characterized by poor survival on environmental surfaces and objects, a
limited range of susceptible anatomic sites (in pediatric gonorrhea: the urethra, vagina, cervix, rectum, throat, and eye), and
presence of the organism at only these sites in those infected.
Thus, an infected individual is by far the most common source
of a new infection.

High-Risk Populations ▶ Older children with gonorrhea tend
to come from family backgrounds of poverty and psychosocial
problems, conditions that increase the risk of sexual abuse by
infected persons.

Mode of Spread ▶ Contamination of a susceptible site by an
infected discharge is required for transmission. Newborns
may acquire the organism from their mothers, either during
delivery or, more rarely, in utero. However, in children outside
the newborn period, sexual contact is the only plausible means
of transmission. The age beyond which the presence of the
organism indicates sexual transmission instead of persistent
perinatal infection is unknown. Infections of the throat or
rectum result from direct inoculation. Transmission by rectal
thermometers, bedding, the much-maligned toilet seat, or by
kissing is highly questionable. In theory, discharge from the
eye could be contagious, but such transmission is extremely
rare. Urine or discharge transferred on the fingers of an infected person has caused disease in the eye.

Incubation Period ▶ The incubation period is usually only
2 to 5 days, and gonococcal conjunctivitis is actually rare in
daycare populations; however, several months' incubation of
perinatally acquired infection has been reported.

DIAGNOSIS

The organism may be presumptively diagnosed by direct
microscopy of a gram-stained specimen. Bacterial culture and
identification of the organism is mandatory, since, at present,
only culture permits subsequent subspecies identification
of the individual organism and possible pinpointing of the

source. The identity of isolates from children should be confirmed by at least two tests that detect different properties of the organism, such as its pattern of fermenting sugars and its antigenic structure. Nonculture methods (e.g., enzyme-linked immunosorbent assay [ELISA], DNA probe, and nucleic acid amplification) for identifying *N. gonorrhoeae* have not been studied adequately in pediatric populations. Because pediatric cases almost always involve the consideration of sexual abuse, careful attention to the chain of custody of the specimen is essential.

TREATMENT

Children with gonorrhea should be treated with a single intramuscular administration of ceftriaxone and an oral dose of azithromycin. Dual therapy is recommended because of antibiotic resistance and because simultaneous infection with *Chlamydia trachomatis* is common in adults. Careful follow-up with test of cure is essential. Hospitalization is required only for management of complications such as severe eye or disseminated infections, or for management of the social situation in sexually abused children. Evaluation for other sexually transmitted infections that may also be present is strongly recommended.

INFECTIOUS PERIOD

The infected person is no longer contagious after 24 hours of receiving effective treatment. Without therapy, the period of contagiousness may last for months.

INFECTION CONTROL

Parental Advice ► If the infection was not acquired at the daycare center or preschool, other parents should not be informed, because the infection is stigmatizing, and the risk of transmission is negligible. Detection of the infection may have forensic implications for the daycare center or preschool.

Vaccine ► None available.

Exclusion from Daycare or Preschool Attendance ► The child may return to daycare the day after effective treatment.

Recommendations for Other Children ▶ The risk of non-sexual transmission to other children is inconsequential. If the child was infected elsewhere, no further measures for control of infection are necessary, but the child may develop emotional and behavioral problems.

Recommendations for Personnel ▶ Handwashing and the use of antibacterial gels and lotions are always important. However, the risk of transmission to the eyes of personnel is small, and the risk of transmission to the genitals is inconsequential.

32

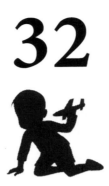

HAEMOPHILUS INFLUENZAE

(Meningitis, Cellulitis, Epiglottitis, Pneumonia, Arthritis)

ChrisAnna M. Mink

SIGNS AND SYMPTOMS

Before the introduction of universal vaccinations, *Haemophilus influenzae* type b (Hib) strains were responsible for 97 percent of the serious invasive infections in children caused by *H. influenzae*. Since introduction of Hib vaccines, the rate of Hib disease in children younger than 5 years of age has declined dramatically to less than 1 per 100,000. In current times, occurrence of invasive Hib infection in a child attending daycare or preschool requires immediate care of the patient, as well as prompt public health intervention.

Systemic or invasive infection begins when *H. influenzae* type b reaches the bloodstream, providing access to many body sites. Invasion is accompanied by a worsening in the child's condition and rapid development of fever. The most common invasive infections are meningitis, cellulitis (or skin and soft tissue infection), epiglottitis, pneumonia, and arthritis. Although *H. influenzae* type b is often isolated from the middle ear, otitis media is not considered a systemic or an invasive infection.

Other non-b strains of *H. influenzae* (a, c–f) and nontypeable strains are a rare cause of invasive infection in healthy children. Nontypeable strains are isolated from the middle ear in about 20 percent of children with ear infections, and may also cause other respiratory infections such as sinusitis, bronchitis, and pneumonia. Infections caused by nontypeable strains of *H. influenzae* and strains with capsular types other than type b generally do not require public health intervention.

CAUSE

The *Haemophilus influenzae* bacterium is a small, gram-negative coccobaccilus. Strains are classified based on the presence of a serologically distinct polysaccharide capsule (capsular types a–f) or on the absence of capsule (nontypeable strains). Type b is the one that is most concerning as an infectious agent in children and the only strain targeted by the vaccine.

SPREAD AND CONTROL

Source of the Organism ▶ *H. influenzae* is a human pathogen, primarily found in the upper respiratory tract. Infection with *H. influenzae*, in the absence of disease, is called colonization or carrier state. Before introduction of the *H. influenzae* type b vaccine in the United States in 1988, up to 5 percent of healthy preschool children carried this germ in their nose and throats. Older children and adults had rates of colonization of about 0.1 percent. Colonization may persist for a few weeks to several months and contributes to the natural acquisition of antibody that protects against invasive disease. Before universal vaccination of infants in the United States, at least a third of all children became carriers at some time before 5 years of age; 1 in 200 to 250 children developed invasive infection. Since 1993 and after the introduction of the vaccine, colonization rates for children have been less than 1 percent and invasive infections have become uncommon in the United States. In countries without Hib vaccines, the occurrence of Hib invasive disease remains elevated.

High-Risk Populations ▶ In the United States, 75 to 90 percent of invasive *H. influenzae* type b infections in children occur before 2 years of age. Unimmunized children younger than 4 years of age, individuals who are immunodeficient or immunocompromised, the elderly, and those who have abnormal or no splenic function (e.g., sickle cell disease) have increased rates of serious, invasive infection caused by *H. influenzae* type b.

Unimmunized children who are younger than 4 years of age and who are siblings or household contacts exposed to a case of invasive *H. influenzae* type b infection are at increased risk of invasive infection. Unimmunized children who are younger than 24 months of age and who are classmates of a case in daycare also may be at slightly increased risk of invasive infection.

Mode of Spread ► *H. influenzae* type b bacteria are found in high concentrations in nasal secretions and occasionally in low concentrations in the saliva of healthy children who are carriers. In nasal secretions, some bacteria live for several hours on nonabsorbent surfaces (e.g., plastic). Spread probably occurs after infected secretions reach the mucous membranes of the nose, eye, or mouth either after coughing or sneezing. Spread also occurs when contaminated objects, such as face cloths or nose wipes, food, toys, or hands, come in contact with the mucous membranes.

Incubation Period ► No incubation period for invasive infection with *H. influenzae* type b has been determined. Clusters of cases, usually within a 60-day period, occur rarely. The long and variable interval between "primary" and "subsequent" cases in both households and daycare suggests they arise more commonly after exposure to children who are carriers than after direct exposure to the first case of active infection.

DIAGNOSIS

The only certain method of diagnosing *H. influenzae* type b infection is by isolation of the organism from a normally sterile body fluid or tissue (e.g., blood and cerebrospinal, pleural, or joint fluid), or from an aspirate of an area of cellulitis. Positive cultures obtained from the throat, ear, or eye (conjunctiva) indicate local, not invasive infection.

TREATMENT

Initial antibiotic treatment of suspected or proven *H. influenzae* type b infections should be administered in an inpatient setting, which permits monitoring for clinical response and possible complications. Until culture results and antibiotic susceptibility tests are known, empiric therapy usually includes a third-generation cephalosporin, because of the ability of these agents to cross the blood-brain barrier and their resistance to β-lactamase activity. Meropenem is an acceptable alternative. In addition to antibiotics, adjunctive and supportive therapies are important in the management of children with invasive Hib disease. Children who have had meningitis should have their hearing tested and should have ongoing monitoring of their development.

INFECTIOUS PERIOD

Intravenous or intramuscular antibiotic therapy of invasive *H. influenzae* type b infection usually suppresses or eradicates colonization in less than 24 hours. Children with invasive Hib disease who receive treatment with agents other than ceftriaxone or cefotaxime (e.g., meropenem or ampicillin) and who are younger than 2 years of age or have susceptible household contacts should receive rifampin for eradication of carriage at the end of their treatment course. In addition, children with invasive Hib infections who are younger than 2 years of age and not fully vaccinated should complete an age-appropriate schedule of *H. influenzae* type b conjugate vaccine starting 1 month after recovery from the invasive infection.

Healthy children and patients who are carriers of *H. influenzae* type b can transmit the bacterium.

INFECTION CONTROL

All home-based and institutional childcare facilities should maintain standard infection control policies and procedures for care of the attendees, staff, and the facility. Policies for required immunizations and for attendance when ill for the children and staff should be clearly outlined and followed.

Following a case of invasive Hib infection, the risk of secondary infection is increased among unimmunized household contacts younger than 4 years of age. Although the risk of secondary infection is also increased among daycare and preschool contacts, the risk is lower than among household contacts. When all daycare and preschool contacts are over the age of 2 years, the occurrence of secondary cases is rare.

Parental Advice ► The parents of children who are in the classroom or in the same group of any child who has invasive *H. influenzae* type b infection should be notified in writing. The notification letter should inform them of (a) the date of the infection, (b) the classroom or group assignment of the case child, (c) the correct name of the germ, and (d) the recommendations for children at the facility. Parents should also be informed of the signs of infection, and of the importance of prompt medical attention and notification of the childcare provider in the event their child becomes ill. Parents should be encouraged to make sure their child is fully immunized with the *H. influenzae* type b conjugate vaccine.

Vaccine ► To prevent invasive *H. influenzae* type b infections, three or four doses of a conjugate vaccine are universally recommended for all infants starting at approximately 2 months of age. Children younger than 5 years of age who have not received the Hib vaccine should receive Hib vaccines following the "catch-up" schedule from the American Academy of Pediatrics and the Advisory Committee for Immunization Practices of the Centers for Disease Control and Prevention (CDC).

Exclusion from Daycare or Preschool Attendance ► Children who have invasive *H. influenzae* type b infection may return to the daycare or preschool once they have received sufficient treatment for eradication of carriage and they are well enough to participate in the program. Most children receiving rifampin prophylaxis will not be contagious after taking the second dose.

Recommendations for Other Children ► When the first case of invasive *H. influenzae* type b infection occurs in a child attending a daycare center or preschool, the patient may well have acquired the infection from siblings, playmates, or other contacts and may not have transmitted the bacteria to classmates. The patient also could have acquired the infection from healthy carriers among their classmates at the childcare center or other contacts. Before universal vaccination, the risk of a second case in the same group of children was estimated to be 0 to 1.3 percent during the first 60 days after the primary case among children younger than 24 months of age. As the risk of a second case is low, antibiotic prophylaxis may not be warranted; however, the children should be monitored carefully for signs and symptoms of infection. The following recommendations apply to children and adult care providers in the same classroom or care group as the child with serious *H. influenzae* type b infection:

- Confirm that the ill child's infection is invasive, such as meningitis, epiglottitis, pneumonia, cellulitis, or bacteremia (not ear, sinus, or conjunctival infection).

- Report confirmed cases to appropriate health department officials (required by law in many states).

- Consult with local health officials, the facility medical advisor, or the patient's physician to develop a recommendation for managing the child's contacts, including those at the facility.

- Generally, antibiotic prophylaxis is not indicated for daycare or preschool classmates after 1 case, especially if all contacts are 24 months of age and older.

  ○ For classmates younger than 4 years of age, all parents should be notified of the illness and informed that the risk among contacts is not significantly increased. In addition, all parents should ensure that their child is completely immunized against Hib.

  ○ If all classmates of the patient are younger than 24 months of age and unvaccinated, the contacts should receive appropriate vaccinations and rifampin prophylaxis should be considered.

Occurrence of a Second Case ▸ A second case in a classroom group is more likely than a single case to indicate the presence of *H. influenzae* type b colonization among children in the classroom group. If a second case occurs within 60 days and incompletely vaccinated children remain in the group, carefully supervised administration of rifampin prophylaxis is recommended. Unimmunized children should receive the *H. influenzae* type b conjugate vaccine according to age-appropriate recommendations.

- Rifampin Prophylaxis. Rifampin is 90 to 95 percent effective in temporarily eradicating *H. influenzae* type b from the nose and throat. *H. influenzae* type b strains resistant to rifampin are uncommon. The efficacy of rifampin prophylaxis in preventing subsequent cases in daycare is unknown. Failures have been reported. Rifampin is a prescription antibiotic that should be given only with sufficient knowledge of the recipient's health status to exclude allergy and conditions that might preclude its use. Consider possible contraindications (e.g., pregnancy, liver disease) and drug interactions. Rifampin turns urine, saliva, and tears an orange color, which can stain clothing and soft contact lenses. Some individuals experience nausea or vomiting or rash while taking rifampin. Rifampin is taken orally for 4 days.

- Most secondary household cases occur within 7 days of hospitalization of the original case, thus, when indicated, antibiotic prophylaxis should be given as soon as possible after diagnosis of the case. In a group setting, prophylaxis is most likely to be effective if given to all group members at the same time. This prevents reacquisition from untreated individuals. All members of the classroom or group are candidates for prophylaxis, including vaccinated children, those older than 24 months, those unexposed or enrolled after the case-patient's illness, and adult caregivers.

- There are no specific recommendations regarding enrollment of new children at a facility after a case of invasive *H. influenzae* type b infection. Children who are eligible for vaccine (2 months of age or older) should have had at least one dose of *H. influenzae* type b conjugate vaccine before starting to attend the facility. If rifampin prophylaxis is to be given, new children who will be assigned to a classroom where there was a case should wait to attend the facility until prophylactic treatment is completed.

Recommendations for Personnel ► Healthy adult caregivers of children in classroom groups with a case of invasive *H. influenzae* type b infection are at extremely low risk of infection. However, up to 7 percent of adult caregivers are Hib carriers when two or more cases occur in a daycare center or preschool classroom. Thus, when rifampin prophylaxis is given to children, it should also be given to their caregivers.

33

HEPATITIS A

Trudy V. Murphy

SIGNS AND SYMPTOMS

Few children younger than 6 years who are infected with the hepatitis A virus (HAV) have symptoms, whereas three quarters of infections among adults are symptomatic. HAV spreads easily among children in childcare settings. Often, the initial clue that HAV transmission is occurring is the report of clinical illness among the adults, either caretakers or family members of the children who are in contact with infected children. Outbreaks can continue without detection for more than a year when childcare management is unaware of this pattern of HAV infections. Typical signs and symptoms found among symptomatic older children are jaundice or yellowing of the skin, dark urine, malaise, and light-colored stools. Diarrhea is a common finding among children, but is uncommon among adults. There is no evidence that HAV causes a persistent infection or progressive liver damage.

CAUSE

The HAV is a small RNA virus. There is only one single strain of hepatitis A virus found worldwide.

SPREAD AND CONTROL

Source of the Organism ▸ Humans are the only source of the HAV. There is no evidence for an animal or inanimate reservoir of the virus.

High-Risk Populations ▸ There are no markers such as age, race, or gender that place a person at higher susceptibility to infection. Exposure is primarily through oral ingestion of fecally contaminated objects or food. Daycare centers and preschools that have children who are not toilet-trained are at higher risk of having HAV transmission than those with only toilet-trained children as clients. Among centers with non-toilet–trained children, those that have lapses in infection-control practice that permit fecal contamination after diaper changing are at greater risk for having HAV transmission than those that maintain scrupulous infection control practices.

Since the institution of hepatitis A vaccination programs in 1999 for children ages 2 to 18 years living in states with a high incidence of disease, there has been a dramatic decrease in the number of reported cases in all ages. In 2006, the Advisory Committee on Immunization Practices recommended routine 2-dose hepatitis A vaccination for all children starting at 12 months of age.

Mode of Spread ▸ Hepatitis A is transmitted primarily by the fecal–oral route, on contaminated hands or objects, in food, or, uncommonly, in water.

Incubation Period ▸ The incubation period is 15 to 50 days.

DIAGNOSIS

As most infections among children are asymptomatic, blood testing for immunity to the virus is the most reliable means of diagnosing HAV infection. A single blood specimen tested for immunoglobulin M (IgM) anti-HAV and immunoglobulin G (IgG) anti-HAV can indicate that an IgM-negative, IgG-negative person has never had the infection and is susceptible and not currently infected. An IgM-positive, IgG-negative result indicates that the person is currently infected or was infected within the past few months. An IgM-positive, IgG-positive result indicates that the person was infected approximately 2 to 6 months ago. An IgM-negative, IgG-positive result indicates that the person was infected more than 6 months ago.

TREATMENT

There is no known effective therapy for HAV infection. Supportive therapy to maintain fluid and caloric intake usually is sufficient, and hospitalization is rarely required.

INFECTIOUS PERIOD

Persons with hepatitis A infection are infectious 2 weeks before onset of the illness and for about 7 to 10 days after the onset of the symptoms. Persons who have no symptoms are also highly infectious. By the time a person is ill enough to seek treatment, he/she usually has passed the period when they are most infectious.

INFECTION CONTROL

Recommendations for Other Children and Personnel and Parental Advice ▶ Because hepatitis A is a disease that is reportable to the health department, and the occurrence of a single symptomatic child, family member of a child in daycare, or adult caretaker often means an outbreak is occurring at the daycare center or preschool, it is important to notify the local health authority. The health authorities are the only ones with the expertise to investigate the situation and make recommendations concerning other children, personnel, and parents of children at the center. Issues such as antibody testing, use of immune serum globulin, and vaccine, and/or closure of the center involve considerable expense and should be approached judiciously. Until the proper authorities can investigate and recommend control measures, parents of children can be taught simple infection control measures to minimize fecal-oral transmission so as to protect family members from further spread; personnel can examine diaper-changing and handwashing practices so as to prevent further spread; and other children can be observed carefully for onset of illness. Finally, the daycare center or preschool must communicate about the situation with each family it serves and assist the authorities with the investigation.

Vaccine ▸ An inactivated HAV vaccine was licensed in 1995. In the summer of 2005, the U.S. Food and Drug Administration licensed the vaccine to be used in children starting at 1 year of age. In 2006, the Advisory Committee on Immunization Practices recommended that all children in the United States be vaccinated to prevent hepatitis A infection starting at 1 year of age. Hepatitis A vaccine after two doses is 94 to 100 percent effective in preventing infection and vaccine protection is estimated to last for at least 20 years.

The vaccine's indications list several other populations in which the vaccine should be used: the vaccine is indicated for high-risk groups (travelers, illicit drug users, men who have sex with men, patients with underlying liver disease). Hepatitis A vaccine is recommended for all employees in child daycare centers and preschools. A combined hepatitis A and hepatitis B vaccine is available and is equally efficacious when compared to either the hepatitis A or hepatitis B vaccine alone. It is recommended that all unimmunized childcare personnel be vaccinated against both hepatitis A and B viruses.

Exclusion from Daycare or Preschool Attendance ▸ Symptomatic children may return to a daycare or preschool setting 10 days after onset of symptoms. Asymptomatic children will be identified in the context of an outbreak, and the epidemiologic circumstances will determine when it is safe for them to return. The outbreak investigators, usually public health authorities, are in the best position to make this decision.

34

HEPATITIS B

Trudy V. Murphy

SIGNS AND SYMPTOMS

Hepatitis B virus (HBV) infection in children causes symptoms in less than 10 percent of cases. When it is symptomatic, the typical signs and symptoms of fatigue, anorexia, jaundice, dark urine, light stools, nausea, vomiting, and abdominal pain are indistinguishable from other causes of hepatitis. The younger a person is at the time of infection, the greater is their risk of developing chronic HBV or life-long infection, which is associated with a substantial risk of cirrhosis, liver failure, and hepatocellular carcinoma later in childhood or as an adult.

CAUSE

HBV is a DNA virus. There are different strains, but in any given geographic location a single strain predominates. Immunity is group-specific, so infection with one subtype usually confers immunity to other subtypes.

SPREAD AND CONTROL

Source of the Organism ▸ The source of infection is a person either newly infected or a person with chronic HBV infection. The virus is found in highest concentrations in blood or in body fluids from blood, e.g., drainage from wounds, sores, or skin conditions, and is found in much lower concentrations in other body fluids such as saliva, urine, or stool.

High-Risk Populations ► In the United States, most preadolescents who are infected with HBV are those born to women with new or chronic infection, or those children who are regularly exposed in the household to persons who have chronic HBV infection. Most hepatitis B acquired from an infected mother at the time of birth can be prevented by vaccinating and giving hepatitis B immune globulin at the time of birth, and by completing the vaccination series. Universal screening for hepatitis B surface antigen (HBsAg) is recommended for all pregnant women, facilitating identification and providing preventive therapies for their at-risk infants. Nevertheless, some women are not screened and their infants fail to receive post-exposure prophylaxis. For those infants or children whose mothers were not screened during pregnancy, reliance on maternal risk history (e.g., immigrant from Asia, Africa, or the Middle East; intravenous drug use; sexual activity with multiple partners) is relatively poor in accurately identifying infected women, and thus would also not identify children in households with persons who have chronic HBV infection.

Mode of Spread ► HBV is transmitted via needle sticks or mucosal exposure to infected blood or other body fluids from a person who is infected with the hepatitis B virus. Transmission can occur in household settings or in institutions for persons with cognitive disabilities, but the risk of transmission in these settings only becomes significant over time with repeated exposures. The mode of transmission in these settings is not fully understood. Shared toothbrushes, drainage from wounds, or aggressive behavior such as biting have been proposed as primary modes of spread. As HBV can survive on environmental surfaces for up to 7 days, environmental contamination could play a role. When institutionalized children with cognitive disabilities have been placed in normal school classrooms, the risk of transmission has been less than 1 percent per year, even with the children with disabilities showing aggressive or self-mutilative behavior and sharing food, eating utensils, and toys they put in their mouths. There has been only one reported instance where transmission occurred in a childcare setting. In that situation, the infected child was engaging in unusually aggressive behavior. In another reported instance, a person with known chronic HBV infection and severe eczema transmitted HBV to a household member but did not transmit the infection to others in a childcare setting, despite being in that setting for a number of months.

Incubation Period ▸ The incubation period ranges from 6 weeks to 6 months.

DIAGNOSIS

Because most infections are asymptomatic, blood testing to detect the virus and antibodies is the most accurate means to diagnose HBV infection. A person with a positive hepatitis B surface antigen (HBsAg) test and a positive test for anti-hepatitis B core (antiHBc) IgM antibody is acutely infected. A person with a positive HBsAg and a positive anti-HBc IgG antibody is a chronic carrier (must be positive for HBsAg 6 months later to confirm this). A person who is hepatitis B surface antibody (anti-HBs) positive has been infected in the past or has been vaccinated and is now immune. A person who is negative for hepatitis B surface antigen (HBsAg), core antibody (anti-HBc) and surface antibody (anti-HBs) is not infected and has not been infected but is susceptible to infection.

TREATMENT

The goal of therapy for chronic HBV infection is to lower the number of viral particles in the blood and to prevent or slow the progression to cirrhosis, liver failure, and hepatocellular carcinoma. A number of antiviral therapies are approved for treatment of chronic hepatitis B infection. Treatment can be associated with significant side effects. The endpoint of treatment remains undefined. Drug resistance and low cure rates have been problematic.

INFECTIOUS PERIOD

Persons are considered infectious if their hepatitis B surface antigen (HBsAg) test is positive. There have been rare reports of persons with a negative HBsAg test but a positive anti-hepatitis

B core (anti-HBc) test who have transmitted HBV, but most persons with this serologic profile are not infectious.

INFECTION CONTROL

Parental Advice ▸ Parents may not know that their child has chronic HBV infection. If the child is known to have chronic HBV infection, a decision about the suitability of childcare can be made in consultation with the child's physician and parents on an individual basis. Parents generally can be informed of the very low risk of transmission of HBV in the daycare setting and steps can be taken to minimize the risk. All parents should ensure their child completes the hepatitis B vaccination series as soon as feasible. Excluding a chronically infected child could be a consideration if the infected child displays aggressive behavior that cannot be controlled or has chronic bleeding or a generalized skin disease. Exclusion would be an option of last resort and, in the case of the deinstitutionalized developmentally challenged child in school classrooms, exclusion is legally indefensible when transmission cannot be demonstrated.

Vaccine ▸ Very effective vaccines to prevent hepatitis B infection are available in a 3- or 4-dose series. Hepatitis B vaccination is recommended for all infants starting at birth and should be a requirement for daycare center or preschool entry. Hepatitis B vaccination for infants and children has resulted in major decreases in hepatitis B infections among children in the United States. A combined hepatitis A and hepatitis B vaccine is available for persons 18 years or older. In previously unimmunized childcare personnel, this combination vaccine is an ideal method of providing protection against both the hepatitis A and B viruses.

Exclusion from Daycare or Preschool Attendance ▸ HBV-infected children need not be excluded from the daycare or preschool setting if they have no aggressive behavior, no generalized skin eruptions, or problems with bleeding. This decision can be made on an individual basis in consultation with the child's physician. Other than the single instance of transmission described earlier, there has been no report of an HBV outbreak in a childcare setting. In transmission studies of deinstitutionalized children with cognitive disabilities whose behaviors are more likely to transmit HBV than children in the normal childcare setting, the risk was extremely low. Exclusion should be considered only after education of parents, personnel, and children on ways to prevent transmission has failed and universal vaccination has not yet occurred. If a child is excluded, then exclusion should last only as long as the child tests positive for HBsAg or the excluding condition remains unresolved.

Recommendations for Other Children ▶ All children attending daycare facilities and preschools should have received a hepatitis B vaccine series unless known to have had past infection. Children should also be taught how to minimize the risk of transmission: don't bite, always put a bandage on cuts and scrapes, and don't share toothbrushes.

Recommendations for Personnel ▶ Personnel are at very low risk of becoming infected by a child and it is suggested that all personnel receive the hepatitis B vaccination. Personnel should be instructed to observe the children for biting or other aggressive behavior, for uncovered cuts or scrapes, and for sharing of toothbrushes. If universal vaccination has not occurred and the behavior continues to be a problem, then the use of vaccine or exclusion of the infected child should be reconsidered by the management of the center. Acute hepatitis B is a reportable condition. Local health authorities are best equipped to assess the situation and to determine if additional control measures are needed.

35

HEPATITIS C

Trudy V. Murphy

SIGNS AND SYMPTOMS

The disease caused by the hepatitis C virus (HCV) is the same as the hepatitis due to hepatitis A virus or hepatitis B virus, although in most cases the signs, symptoms, and liver function test abnormalities are not as severe. Persistent infection is more common with hepatitis C disease and develops in approximately 85 percent of infected patients. Chronic active hepatitis develops in 60 to 70 percent of those infected with hepatitis C and cirrhosis develops in approximately 20 percent. Mother-to-child transmission of HCV has become the leading source of HCV infection in children.

CAUSE

The hepatitis C virus is an RNA virus.

SPREAD AND CONTROL

Source of the Organism ▸ The source of infection is a person with chronic HCV infection.

High-Risk Populations ▸ The highest rates of HCV infection occur in persons with repeated needle-stick exposure to blood or blood products. Intravenous drug users and hemophiliacs have a seroprevalence (documented infection rate by blood testing) of 60 to 90 percent. Hemodialysis patients have a 20 percent seroprevalence, household and sexual contacts of infected persons, a 1 to 10 percent seroprevalence, and health care workers, a 1 percent seroprevalence. Perinatal transmission has been documented in approximately 5 percent of infants born to HCV-infected or pregnant women who are infected with both HCV and HIV.

Mode of Spread ► Infection is spread primarily by needle-stick exposure to blood and blood products from a person with HCV infection, or from mother to infant at the time of birth, or possibly, intrauterine infection. For many infected children, no specific source for their infection is identified. There have been no reports of transmission of HCV in childcare settings.

Incubation Period ► The incubation period of HCV averages 6 to 7 weeks.

DIAGNOSIS

Diagnostic blood tests documenting antibodies to the hepatitis C virus are available. This is a two-stage test: an enzyme-linked immunosorbent antibody assay (ELISA), which, if positive, is confirmed by a test for specific HCV RNA. Within 5 to 6 weeks after the onset of disease, 80 percent of patients will have detectable antibodies. Because viral RNA may be detected only intermittently, detection of the presence of HCV RNA by polymerase chain reaction (PCR) in at least 2 serum samples at least 3 months apart is recommended during the first year of life, or testing can be conducted for antibodies against HCV after 18 months of age in any child born to a mother with HCV infection.

TREATMENT

There are an increasing number of antiviral agents being developed for the treatment of hepatitis C. Treatment responses vary with the infecting hepatitis C genotype, viral load, and host genetics. Recombinant interferon alone and in combination with ribavirin are available and have been licensed for the treatment of chronically infected patients. All patients with hepatitis C should be evaluated by a specialist in treating hepatitis C and should receive hepatitis A and B vaccines to prevent other and compounding sources of liver damage.

INFECTIOUS PERIOD

All persons with antibody to HCV or detection of the hepatitis C RNA in the blood are considered infectious.

INFECTION CONTROL

Exclusion from Daycare or Preschool Attendance, Recommendations for Other Children and Personnel, and Parental Advice ▸ Until there are data demonstrating that transmission of HCV occurs in a daycare or preschool setting, no exclusion of children with HCV infection is indicated. To date, no outbreaks of HCV have been reported in these settings, nor have there been case reports suggesting possible disease transmission in a daycare or preschool setting. Adherence to scrupulous standard precautions to prevent transmission of bloodborne pathogens in this setting should prevent transmission of HCV.

Vaccine ▸ None available.

36

HERPES SIMPLEX VIRUS

(Gingivostomatitis)

Richard J. Whitley

SIGNS AND SYMPTOMS

The herpes simplex virus causes a wide spectrum of diseases ranging from asymptomatic and benign infections, such as fever blisters, to life-threatening diseases, such as neonatal disseminated herpes infection and herpes simplex encephalitis. Infections caused by herpes simplex virus in individuals who are immunocompromised can be severe. The most common childhood manifestation of herpes simplex infections are herpes simplex gingivostomatitis, a disease of the mouth and throat characterized by crusty ulcerative lesions in the mouth in association with fever and severe pain. The oral pain can lead to hospitalization because of inadequate oral fluid intake.

Other childhood manifestations of herpes simplex infections include herpes simplex eye infection (keratoconjunctivitis), neonatal herpes simplex virus infection presenting within the first 4 weeks of life, and herpes simplex central nervous system infection (encephalitis). Children who are immunocompromised can have unappreciated older infection reactivate and result in severe and progressive orofacial disease.

Patients with herpes simplex infections are most contagious to other individuals when skin or mucous membrane lesions are present.

CAUSE

Herpes simplex virus consists of two serotypes: herpes simplex type 1, which generally causes infections above the belt, and herpes simplex type 2, which generally causes infections below the belt, although this distinction is becoming less common. All members of the herpes virus family are large DNA viruses.

SPREAD AND CONTROL

Source of the Organism ► The virus is found only in infectious secretions of individuals actively replicating the herpes simplex virus. Sites from which the herpes simplex virus can be retrieved are vesicular lesions, the oropharynx during gingivostomatitis, tissue obtained at biopsy of individuals with severely progressive disease, and from the genital tract during episodes of recurrent genital herpes. Recently, by polymerase chain reaction (PCR) testing that detects the viral DNA, the herpes simplex virus DNA has been detected in the saliva of 1 percent of normal healthy individuals and in genital secretions in the absence of detectable lesions.

High-Risk Populations ► High-risk populations include individuals with compromised immune function and babies born to women who have a genital herpetic infection at delivery.

Mode of Spread ► Transmission of the herpes simplex virus is by direct and intimate personal contact. The virus has not been known to be transmitted from inanimate objects to human beings. Intimate personal human contact is the only mechanism known today for transmission of this infection.

Incubation Period ► The incubation period is from 3 to 5 days.

DIAGNOSIS

Infections caused by the herpes simplex virus are usually diagnosed by clinical manifestations. In most individuals, the vesicular rash is diagnostic; however, the virus can be isolated in cell culture systems. Under unusual circumstances, the diagnosis of neonatal herpes simplex infection and herpes simplex encephalitis is often more difficult. Excretion of the virus from peripheral sites in such individuals is often rare, and, therefore, obtaining tissue for isolation of the virus is essential. Detection of viral DNA in the cerebrospinal fluid by PCR testing is the best diagnostic approach when the test is performed by a reputable laboratory.

TREATMENT

The only forms of herpes simplex virus infections that require therapy are those involving the newborn, children with herpes simplex encephalitis, and the immunocompromised child with recurrent herpes simplex infections. Acyclovir is the treatment of choice, and the only formulation currently licensed for use in children is that for intravenous administration. Some physicians treat gingivostomatitis with oral acyclovir, famciclovir, or valacyclovir.

INFECTIOUS PERIOD

The duration of infectivity is approximately 4 to 5 days once intravenous acyclovir has been started. In the absence of therapy, however, infectivity can persist for as long as 3 weeks.

INFECTION CONTROL

Parental Advice ▶ There is little likelihood that this infection will be transmitted from one child to another.

Vaccine ▶ None available.

Exclusion from Daycare or Preschool Attendance ▶ The child should not attend the daycare center or preschool until the skin lesions are scabbed.

Recommendations for Other Children ▶ Once a child is infected, avoid person-to-person contact and contact with vesicles. To accomplish such a goal, existing vesicles can be covered.

Recommendations for Personnel ▶ Strict handwashing and the use of gloves when changing wound dressings and/or manipulating infected skin will prevent transmission of this virus. Personnel with recurrent herpes labialis (fever blisters) should cover their lesions until crusted and be educated to avoid person-to-person contact and touching of and/or contact with vesicular lesions.

37

HUMAN IMMUNODEFICIENCY VIRUS INFECTION AND ACQUIRED IMMUNODEFICIENCY SYNDROME

Gwendolyn B. Scott

SIGNS AND SYMPTOMS

Infection with human immunodeficiency virus type-1 (HIV-1) results in a progressive deterioration of the immune system, ultimately leading to opportunistic infections, malignancies, and other conditions that represent the spectrum of illnesses comprising the acquired immunodeficiency syndrome (AIDS). In the United States between 1992 and 2009, 5,340 children with AIDS were reported to the Centers for Disease Control and Prevention (CDC).

The majority of these children have acquired HIV infection through mother-to-infant transmission at birth. It is estimated that approximately 7,000 women with HIV infection deliver an infant in the United States yearly. In the absence of antiretroviral therapy, between 20 and 30 percent of HIV-infected pregnant women will transmit HIV to their infants. Since 1994, however, the use of anti-HIV antibiotics that prevent mother-to-child transmission, in addition to other potent antiretroviral drugs, have significantly decreased the risk of transmission of HIV and the number of children with perinatally acquired

200

AIDS. During infancy and early childhood, many HIV-infected children will attend daycare or preschool.

HIV infection in children is a chronic multisystem disease characterized by a wide range of complications and conditions. Prior to the availability of highly active anti-HIV antiretroviral therapies, between 10 and 20 percent of children developed progressive disease with significant immune suppression during the first 2 years of life, with a survival of less than 4 years. The remainder of children had a variable clinical course with a median survival of 8 years. However, earlier identification, diagnosis, and aggressive antiretroviral treatment of HIV infection in children have decreased early complications and have prolonged survival.

The clinical course of HIV infection has changed significantly with the availability of these highly active antiretroviral therapies. There are children who acquired HIV infection at birth who have survived into their thirties. Early diagnosis, reduction of viral load, preservation of the immune system, and compliance with antiretroviral therapy are all factors that influence outcome.

In untreated children with perinatal HIV infection, common early clinical manifestations include failure to thrive or wasting; chronic or recurrent diarrhea without specific cause; generalized lymphadenopathy, hepatosplenomegaly and parotitis; persistent or recurrent thrush or oral candidiasis; and a variety of recurrent infections including otitis media, pneumonia, and meningitis, usually of bacterial origin but also caused by viral, fungal, and parasitic pathogens.

Central nervous system involvement with HIV may present in the infant or young child as developmental delay or loss of developmental milestones. Progressive encephalopathy occurs in about 10 percent of infected children and is usually associated with significant immune deficiency, failure to thrive, spasticity, poor head growth, and evidence of brain atrophy and/or calcifications documented by computed tomography (CT) scanning of the brain. This condition is much less common in children who are diagnosed early and treated with highly active antiretroviral drugs. Older children may manifest learning disabilities or attention deficit disorders. Thus, developmental testing is an important part of routine care so these conditions can be detected early and interventions can be prescribed. Heart, liver, and kidney abnormalities also occur in some children. Malignancies, particularly non-Hodgkin's lymphoma, occur in about 2 percent of HIV-infected children.

AIDS is the "late stage" of infection with HIV. The definition of AIDS, which has been revised several times, includes the presence of opportunistic infection, certain malignancies, recurrent serious bacterial infections, a specific lung infection called lymphoid interstitial pneumonia in children under 13 years of age, and low levels of CD4-positive lymphocytes (<200 cells/mm3) in adults and adolescents. Separate disease classification systems have been developed for both children and adults that relate clinical and immunologic status and describe the spectrum of disease.

Pneumonia caused by *Pneumocystis jiroveci* is the most frequently described opportunistic infection in AIDS. Other common opportunistic infections include candida esophagitis, disseminated cytomegalovirus infection, and disseminated mycobacterial infection, most often caused by *Mycobacterium avium* complex. Both pulmonary and nonpulmonary tuberculosis are increasingly common problems, particularly among adults in selected populations. In some areas, tuberculosis and tuberculosis resistant to multiple drugs in people with AIDS has become a significant public health problem.

CAUSE

HIV is an RNA retrovirus not known to infect other animals naturally. Humans are the only known reservoir of HIV. Two major types of HIV have been identified: HIV-1 and HIV-2. Although both subtypes have been associated with AIDS and related clinical syndromes, HIV-1 has been the predominant cause of disease in the world. HIV-2 infection is more commonly seen in western African countries and is extremely rare in the United States.

SPREAD AND CONTROL

Source of the Organism ▶ Humans are the only known reservoir of HIV.

High-Risk Populations ▶ In the United States, HIV infection and AIDS primarily occur in young adults. Adults (and adolescents) currently at highest risk of acquiring HIV infection include men who have sex with men (homosexual or bisexual males), people who inject drugs or use crack cocaine (the latter because of its association with multiple sex partners), and men and women who have multiple sex partners (some of whom may be at high risk). Approximately 1 to 2 percent of all cases of AIDS reported in the United States have occurred in children or adolescents. Children at highest risk for HIV infection are those born to women who are infected. The highest risk for women is injection of drugs, use of crack cocaine, having multiple sex partners, or being the sex partner of a man at high risk. Infants and children may also become infected through breastfeeding, premastication of food, or sexual abuse by an individual who is HIV-infected. Children or adults who have clotting factor disorders (including classic hemophilia) and who received clotting factor therapy before the mid-1980s are also at high risk of HIV infection and AIDS. Major improvements have been made in the safety of clotting factor concentrates since the mid-1980s, and people with hemophilia not infected before 1986 are no longer at high risk of HIV infection through that route because all donated blood is now screened.

Mode of Spread ▶ HIV infection is acquired through (a) sexual contact with an infected person, whether homosexual or heterosexual; (b) direct inoculation of infectious blood or tissue through use of contaminated needles during intravenous drug injection, a mucous membrane exposure, penetrating injury with a needle or sharp object containing infected blood, tissue or organ transplantation, or, rarely, through receipt of a blood transfusion; and (c) perinatal transmission from an infected woman to her fetus in utero or at delivery to her infant, or postnatally during breastfeeding. For children with HIV in the United States, perinatal transmission accounts for over 95 percent of cases. Significant decreases in perinatal HIV infection have been observed in the United States and Europe following the use of antiretroviral therapy in pregnant women and their infants to reduce transmission of HIV. In the United States, the risk of perinatal transmission is between 1 and 2 percent in women receiving antiretroviral therapy in combination with other antiretroviral drugs.

Transmission by other means such as through food or water, contaminated objects, or casual contact in a household, workplace, childcare, or school setting has not been documented to occur. Several studies of individuals living in households with HIV-infected adults or children have shown no transmission and include 300 children of differing ages followed for more than 1,700 person years. Independent of these studies, there are only six case reports of household transmission of HIV involving children. In most of these cases, the means of transmission is unknown, but percutaneous or intravenous exposure to blood from the infected household contact is possible.

Biting is a common behavior in young children. HIV has been isolated from saliva of some infected persons, but transmission of HIV by bites is rare and has occurred only in association with blood-tinged saliva in the wound. The actual risk of transmission of HIV through biting is thought to be very low. Fluids implicated in the transmission of HIV infection include blood, vaginal secretions, semen, and breast milk.

Incubation Period ► In adults, an acute self-limited illness caused by HIV may occur within a few weeks after infection. Onset of chronic illness usually occurs years after infection, with approximately half of infected adults diagnosed with AIDS 10 years after infection. In children with perinatally acquired infection, illness often becomes apparent during the first or second year of life, although it may occur years later. With other routes of infection (e.g., transfusion), clinical illness and a diagnosis of AIDS may not occur for years.

DIAGNOSIS

The diagnosis of symptomatic HIV infection and AIDS is based on the clinical, blood antibody tests, and immunologic

findings and exclusion of other causes for the immunodeficiency. The presence of certain clinical conditions or opportunistic infections may suggest a diagnosis of HIV infection.
Serologic tests for HIV infection are highly sensitive and
specific if performed by a reliable laboratory. Confirmation
is essential. In a child 2 years of age or older, HIV infection
is diagnosed by an HIV antibody test that is repeatedly positive and confirmed by a Western blot assay or an immunofluorescence test. Before 24 months of age, diagnosis is more
complex because a positive HIV antibody test may only reflect
a maternal antibody that was transferred to her baby during
pregnancy. The standard test for diagnosis of HIV infection in
infants and children under 24 months of age is the polymerase
chain reaction (PCR) for detection of the actual human immunodeficiency virus. The sensitivity of PCR for diagnosis
of HIV is greater than 95 percent by 6 weeks of age. The HIV
PCR can also be used for diagnosis in this age group. Consent
for testing the infant or child for HIV should be obtained from
the parent or legal guardian prior to testing.

TREATMENT

Children with HIV infection need close medical supervision
with monitoring of their clinical, neurologic, developmental,
and immunologic status. Most infants and children with
HIV infection are seen at 3- to 6-month intervals depending
on their clinical status. The child with HIV infection should
receive routine childhood care, including vaccinations, and
should be evaluated promptly if infection or fever occurs.
Therapy of HIV infection includes antiretroviral therapy and
prophylaxis against *P. jirovecii* and other infections.

The American Academy of Pediatrics and the CDC have
published recommendations for immunization of children
with HIV infection against other diseases, and current recommendations should be consulted. Briefly, both symptomatic and asymptomatic children with HIV infection should
receive diphtheria, tetanus, acellular pertussis, inactivated
polio, *Haemophilus influenzae* type b conjugate, conjugated
pneumococcal and meningococcal vaccines, and hepatitis A
and B vaccines following the routine immunization schedule.

In general, live viral (e.g., oral polio [OPV]) and bacterial (e.g., bacillus Calmette–Guérin [BCG]) vaccines should not be given. There are no safety or efficacy data available regarding administration of live attenuated rotavirus vaccine to HIV-infected infants. Because measles can cause severe or fatal illness in children infected with severe HIV disease, measles, mumps, and rubella vaccines are recommended for those HIV-infected children who are not severely immunocompromised. Varicella vaccine should be considered only for HIV-infected children with CD4 percentage of 15 percent or greater. Inactivated influenza vaccine should be given to children 6 months of age or older annually. As children with symptomatic HIV infection may have a poor immunologic response to vaccines, these children should be considered candidates for post-exposure prophylaxis (e.g., immunoglobulin, varicella-zoster immune globulin) if exposed to diseases for which this is available.

Prompt diagnosis and aggressive treatment of opportunistic infections, maintenance of nutritional status, developmental assessment, and good supportive care are important elements of ongoing medical follow-up.

INFECTIOUS PERIOD

Because HIV establishes a chronic infection, an infected person is presumably infectious throughout life. The degree of transmissibility of HIV may vary with the stage of infection and the viral load (number of HIV RNA copies per milliliter) in blood.

INFECTION CONTROL

Parental Advice ► As the risk of transmission of HIV infection among children in a childcare setting is only hypothetical, there is no urgent need to inform parents about the attendance of an infected child at a center. In lieu of special notice, it may be preferable to provide parents with general information about management of infectious diseases, including HIV, before a specific instance arises.

Vaccine ► No effective vaccine for prevention of HIV is currently available.

Post-Exposure Prophylaxis for HIV ► The risk for transmission in health care workers exposed to HIV-infected blood following a needle-stick injury is 0.3 percent and is 0.09 percent following a mucous membrane exposure. There are no large-scale studies available in children who have been exposed to discarded needles in parks, playgrounds, or on the street, but the risk is likely to be small. In the event of such an exposure or an exposure of a child or adult to the blood of an HIV-infected person, the wound or area involved should be washed thoroughly with soap and water and the child or adult referred immediately to his or her physician or the closest emergency room. In some instances, post-exposure prophylaxis with antiretroviral therapy is warranted and should be started as soon as possible following an injury.

Exclusion from Daycare or Preschool Attendance ► HIV-infected children should be allowed to attend daycare centers and schools and allowed to participate in all activities to the extent that their health permits. Attendance at a daycare center should be decided on an individual basis by qualified persons, including the child's physician. Factors to be considered include the type of care the child will receive and whether the infected child would be at significant risk of being exposed to serious infectious diseases. Although the risk of transmission of HIV from one infant or child to another in a childcare setting is unmeasurable and highly improbable based on known means of transmission, it has been a major consideration in all discussions about including HIV-infected children in these settings. In general, young children who have open skin lesions should not be in a childcare setting with other small children. Because of neurologic impairment and developmental delays with HIV infection, decisions about appropriate care settings should be based on developmental stage rather than chronologic age. Periodic reassessment of the child is urged. The American Academy of Pediatrics publishes current recommendations to provide a guide for evaluation of children in this setting. In addition, other infectious conditions in HIV-infected children should be evaluated to determine whether they pose a risk to other children or adults in the care setting. Preschool programs should develop policies to inform all parents when a highly infectious illness, such as measles, chickenpox, parvovirus B19 infection (fifth disease), tuberculosis, or cryptosporidiosis or other acute diarrhea, occurs in a child, so families can take appropriate measures to protect their immunodeficient children.

Recommendations for Other Children ▶ Based on studies of HIV-infected children and adults that have shown no transmission of HIV in a family setting, HIV is highly unlikely to be transmitted from one child to another in a daycare center or preschool. No special precautions are warranted; therefore, admission or continued attendance of an HIV-infected child should be based on a careful case-by-case review as recommended above. Screening of children for HIV infection in a childcare setting before admission or after a child in the center is found to be infected is not justifiable.

Recommendations for Personnel ▶ Because a child may not be known to be infected with HIV (or other bloodborne infectious agents such as hepatitis B virus), all daycare centers and preschools should adopt reasonable policies and procedures for managing accidents, such as a nosebleed, for all students, and for cleaning and disinfecting surfaces contaminated with blood. Gloves should be used if readily available, but direct contact with blood can also be avoided by using several thicknesses of paper towels or folded cloths. Blood-contaminated surfaces should be cleaned and disinfected with freshly prepared chlorine bleach solution (1:10 dilution). Gloves do not need to be used for feeding a child or wiping secretions that do not contain visible blood; they should be used, however (in addition to careful handwashing), for changing diapers that contain bloody stools. Good handwashing is fundamental in prevention of HIV and other infectious diseases. All personnel should have knowledge of appropriate infection-control procedures and have access to necessary supplies. The Occupational Safety and Health Administration (OSHA) has published regulations regarding education of employees and routine procedures for handling blood and bloody fluids.

Personnel who are directly involved with the care of an HIV-infected child in a childcare setting and who have a need to know should be informed of that fact and should be instructed about the need to respect and maintain the rights of the child and family to privacy and confidentiality of the information; the minimum number of persons necessary should be informed. If medical records are maintained, confidentiality must be assured.

HIV-Infected Personnel ► The American Academy of Pediatrics has stated that HIV-infected adults do not pose a risk of infection to children in childcare settings if they do not have open or exudative skin lesions or other medical conditions that would allow contact with potentially infectious (i.e., bloody) fluids. HIV-infected personnel who have other infectious conditions (e.g., active pulmonary or laryngeal tuberculosis, acute diarrhea, or herpetic whitlow) that may be transmitted to others in the childcare setting should be evaluated to determine appropriate management and whether temporary or permanent exclusion is warranted. Immunocompromised adults may be highly susceptible to the infectious agents that young children attending daycare centers or preschools are likely to have, and they should seek advice from their physician about the advisability of such work and what precautions are recommended.

38

INFECTIOUS MONONUCLEOSIS

Ciro V. Sumaya

SIGNS AND SYMPTOMS

Most infections by this virus occur mainly in young children and produce no problems (i.e., they are asymptomatic). In some instances, at a frequency that is not very clear, an infection can produce infectious mononucleosis. This illness consists of a typical clinical picture with fever, tiredness, enlarged neck lymph nodes, inflamed throat and tonsils, and enlargement of abdominal organs (liver and/or spleen). The clinical illness may last 1 to 2 or more weeks.

Sometimes, significant complications can occur during the infectious mononucleosis episode and involve the respiratory tract (pneumonia, severe airway obstruction), nervous system (seizures, meningoencephalitis, nerve palsies), and blood system (decline in platelets and anemia), among others. However, virtually all cases have a transient course with complete resolution and no aftereffects. It is also believed that this virus can cause illnesses characterized by isolated manifestations such as inflamed throats or pneumonia instead of an infectious mononucleosis episode.

CAUSE

Epstein–Barr virus (EBV), the cause of infectious mononucleosis, is a DNA virus.

SPREAD AND CONTROL

Source of the Organism ► It is believed that this virus is present in saliva and therefore can be transmitted through contact that permits salival exchange.

High-Risk Populations ► The virus spreads mainly among children, presumably more rapidly in closed or overcrowded conditions. Why an infection with this virus usually produces no ill effects in young children, while in young adults it is quite likely to produce the infectious mononucleosis syndrome, is unclear. It also seems that if one child in a family develops infectious mononucleosis, there is a greater chance for another child in the family to develop that illness even after a long lapse in time following the initial case. Children with special problems with their immune system or those who have recently received organ or bone marrow transplants are at greater risk for experiencing a serious disease with an infectious mononucleosis episode or other manifestations from their EBV infection.

Mode of Spread ► It is believed that the virus is transmitted through salival exchange. The transmission of EBV via blood products with the subsequent development of an infectious mononucleosis–like illness is quite uncommon.

Incubation Period ► The incubation period of infectious mononucleosis is usually quite long, 5 to 7 weeks after exposure. The incubation period seems to be a few weeks shorter if the exposure to EBV was via a blood transfusion.

DIAGNOSIS

The diagnosis is made by the presence of the following triad of findings: (a) typical signs and symptoms as mentioned above, (b) a blood count showing an increased number of lymphocytes and atypical lymphocyte formation, and (c) a blood antibody test indicating the presence of heterophil antibodies or specific EBV antibodies reflecting an acute infection. In very young children (under 4 years old), a heterophil response may not be detected, necessitating the testing for specific EBV antibodies to confirm the diagnosis.

TREATMENT

Simple measures to reduce or alleviate the signs and symptoms, such as antipyretics to decrease the fever, reduction of activity, and bed rest for the malaise, are commonly recommended for the patient with infectious mononucleosis. Contact sports should be avoided during the time the spleen is felt to be enlarged. Corticosteroids are sometimes administered when the patient has significant complications or an otherwise severe clinical course. The efficacy of the corticosteroids in this condition, however, is still not well documented. The few patients who may develop pronounced respiratory obstruction because of immense tonsillar inflammation may receive an emergency tonsillectomy or require ventilatory support. An antiviral medication, acyclovir, does reduce the amount of EBV in salival excretions of patients with infectious mononucleosis, but does not significantly alter the signs, symptoms, or course of the disease.

INFECTIOUS PERIOD

The length of infectivity is quite unclear, because patients with infectious mononucleosis or other forms of acute EBV infections may excrete the virus intermittently in their saliva for many months, if not years, following their infection. It is presumed, though, that the amount of virus in the saliva during the acute episode of infectious mononucleosis or other form of EBV infection is at its peak and, therefore, more likely to be transmittable to close contacts. In comparison to later in the disease or after resolution of the illness, there are progressively decreasing amounts of virus present.

INFECTION CONTROL

Parental Advice ▸ The parent (or physician) should notify the center supervisor about the diagnosis. An assurance can be provided that this illness is not easily spread (i.e., the development of a second case or more cases of infectious mononucleosis in the center that are related to contact with the initial case should be a rare event).

Vaccine ▶ An experimental vaccine is being tested but is not available for general use.

Exclusion from Daycare or Preschool Attendance ▶ The child should probably be removed from the childcare setting during the period of time that he or she feels ill and unable to tolerate much general activity. In most cases, this is about 1 to 2 weeks.

Recommendations for Other Children ▶ There are no specific recommendations for other children in the center other than the adherence to common hygienic practices such as the washing of hands when potentially contaminated with human secretions and the avoidance of mouthing of toys or mouth-to-mouth kissing.

Recommendations for Personnel ▶ There are no specific recommendations other than the adherence to common hygienic practices as noted. The risk of significant problems to a pregnant woman (and her unborn child) from exposure to a child with infectious mononucleosis is considered extremely low.

39

INFLUENZA

(Flu)

Scott A. Halperin

SIGNS AND SYMPTOMS

Influenza virus causes a spectrum of clinical symptoms that make up the "flu syndrome." In the first several days of infection, fever, headache, myalgias, and chills are prominent. Burning and tearing of the eyes also occur during this period. Respiratory symptoms, including cough and runny nose, are present at the onset but become more noticeable after the third day when the fever and systemic manifestations subside. Respiratory symptoms persist for 3 or 4 days, although the cough may persist for 1 to 2 weeks.

Influenza infections occur in epidemics during the winter months. The spread is rapid through a community, with widespread absenteeism from work and school. Muscle and joint pain and headaches are typically seen in older children and adults. Younger school-aged children and preschool-aged children typically have milder disease, although the fever may be higher. Infants and toddlers have rates of hospitalization similar to the elderly. Secondary complications occur frequently during influenza epidemics, although these are less common in children. Primary viral pneumonia due to influenza virus can occur, as well as secondary bacterial pneumonia due to *Streptococcus pneumoniae, Haemophilus influenzae,* or *Staphylococcus aureus.* In young children, croup and bronchitis may occur due to infection with influenza virus. A rare but serious complication of an influenza virus infection in children is Reye's syndrome.

CAUSE

Three virus types are known: influenza A, influenza B, and influenza C. The influenza virus is an RNA virus. The unique characteristic of influenza virus is the frequency with which it changes its antigenicity. With influenza A, antigenic variation occurs on an almost annual basis; small changes (antigenic drift) occur each year which thus means that immunity to this virus is not reliable because the virus has changed. This allows for annual epidemics and the need for new vaccines each year. Large changes (antigenic shift) are associated with more severe and widespread disease (pandemics) such as occurred with the H1N1 swine origin strain in 2009. Variation also occurs with influenza B but has not been shown with influenza C virus.

SPREAD AND CONTROL

Source of the Organism ▸ Influenza virus is found in respiratory secretions of infected individuals.

High-Risk Populations ▸ Because of continual change of the antigenic composition of the virus, individuals may continue to be susceptible to influenza virus infection from year to year. Children at high risk include those with chronic lung disease, such as moderate to severe asthma, cystic fibrosis, and bronchopulmonary dysplasia. Severe disease also occurs in children with significant cardiac anomalies, immunosuppressed children, and children with hemoglobinopathies (including sickle cell disease), diabetes, chronic renal failure, and metabolic diseases. Healthy infants younger than 1 year of age have higher rates of hospitalization for influenza illness comparable to those of the elderly.

Mode of Spread ▸ Influenza is spread from person to person by direct contact with infected secretions or via large- or small-droplet aerosols.

Incubation Period ► One to 3 days.

DIAGNOSIS

Influenza virus infection may be diagnosed by culture of the virus in egg or tissue culture. The virus also can be detected directly in secretions from the nose and throat by using direct or indirect immunofluorescent tests or enzyme immunoassay tests. Nucleic acid detection such as polymerase chain reaction (PCR) is more sensitive and is increasingly replacing culture and other rapid tests for the diagnosis of influenza. However, during an epidemic, the diagnosis is usually made clinically.

TREATMENT

Most children with influenza virus infection do not require specific therapy. In children at risk for severe or complicated disease due to underlying conditions, antiviral treatment is recommended. Oseltamivir is effective against both influenza A and B viruses and is available as an oral suspension approved for use in children 1 year of age and older; treatment is best started within 2 days of symptom onset. Zanamivir, an inhaled antiviral medicine, is approved for use in children 7 years of age and older. To be effective, it is best started within 2 days of symptom onset. Amantadine and rimantadine therapy have been shown to be effective in reducing the symptoms caused by influenza A virus only, particularly if started very early in the course of the illness. Therapy is usually continued for 3 to 5 days. Aspirin and aspirin-containing products should be avoided due to their association with the subsequent development of Reye's syndrome in influenza patients. Hospitalization is only required for those with severe illness.

INFECTIOUS PERIOD

The virus may be found in respiratory secretions for 6 days prior to the onset of symptoms until 7 days after the symptoms began for influenza A virus, and from 1 day before to 2 weeks after onset of symptoms for influenza B virus infections.

INFECTION CONTROL

Parental Advice ▶ Parents should be advised that childcare attendees and all of their family members and contacts should be immunized against influenza annually. Parents should be advised that an influenza outbreak is occurring and should be instructed to monitor for any complications or severe infection. Aspirin or aspirin-containing products should be avoided during influenza infections because of the association with Reye's syndrome.

Vaccine ▶ The influenza vaccine is recommended for all children 6 months of age and older. The vaccine is particularly important for high risk children with chronic lung disease, moderate to severe asthma, bronchopulmonary dysplasia, cystic fibrosis, significant cardiac disease, children receiving immunosuppressive therapy, children with hemoglobinopathies, diabetes, human immunodeficiency virus infection, and individuals with rheumatoid arthritis or Kawasaki's disease on long-term aspirin therapy. Immunization is now recommended for all adults in the United States. Immunization of close contacts of severely immunocompromised children is of particular importance because these children may have a suboptimal antibody response to the vaccine. Immunization of close contacts of infants from birth to 6 months of age is also recommended because these infants are at highest risk of influenza-related hospitalization but are too young to receive the vaccine. Influenza vaccine should be encouraged for all daycare attendees, staff, and household contacts as part of the universal influenza immunization program. A live-virus vaccine that can be given intranasally and which has been demonstrated to be effective in children is available and may facilitate recommendations for universal use of influenza vaccines in children.

Exclusion from Daycare or Preschool Attendance ▶ Once influenza is introduced into a childcare facility, most children will have been exposed before the onset of symptoms. Therefore, exclusion of a child with influenza infection is not necessary, and attendance should be based on the condition of the child. However, it is not uncommon for childcare facilities to close during an influenza epidemic because of high absenteeism among staff and high absenteeism among children who are too sick to attend.

Recommendations for Other Children ► Children with symptoms of influenza should be monitored for any complications that would require examination by the family physician.

Recommendations for Personnel ► Influenza virus infection is typically spread from children to their caregivers. The infection spreads rapidly through the facility, and most susceptible individuals will become infected. As part of the universal influenza immunization program, it is particularly important that all daycare and preschool providers receive a yearly influenza vaccine. Careful handwashing and attention to respiratory secretions may diminish the spread of infection.

40

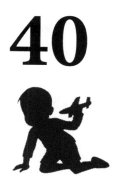

MENINGOCOCCUS

(Bacteremia, Meningitis, Arthritis)

Eugene D. Shapiro

SIGNS AND SYMPTOMS

The most common manifestations of illness caused by *Neisseria meningitidis* in children are central nervous system infection (meningitis, bloodstream infection with or without septic shock), arthritis, and pneumonia, any of which may occur alone or in combination with one or more of the others. In children with meningitis, fever usually develops, and they may have a stiff neck and often become irritable or lethargic. This condition may progress to coma. Children with meningococcal sepsis (with or without meningitis) may develop a characteristic rash that consists of small, flat, red spots (petechiae) that do not blanch when pressed on the extremities and/or on the trunk. Occasionally, patients develop an overwhelming illness with rapidly progressive septic shock, often associated with a hemorrhagic rash (purpura fulminans).

CAUSE

Meningococcal infections are caused by a type of bacteria, *N. meningitidis*. These bacteria are divided into more than ten different serogroups and most infections in the United States are caused by serogroups B, C, and Y.

SPREAD AND CONTROL

Source of the Organism ▸ The organism is part of the normal bacterial flora of the human mouth. It is usually carried in the nasopharynx (the throat). At any given time, 5 to 10 percent of healthy people harbor the bacteria in their throat. However, in a daycare center in which one case of an invasive meningococcal infection has occurred, up to 50 percent or more of the children and adults in the group may be colonized with the organism.

High-Risk Populations ▸ Children with deficiencies of antibody or complement or who have abnormalities or absence of their spleens are at increased risk of infection. Although both children and adults who are exposed may be at risk, younger children are at the greatest risk.

Mode of Spread ▸ The organism is spread by respiratory droplets or by direct oral contact with someone who is colonized with the bacteria. Although many people worry about the organism spreading from an infected child to others, in most instances other children in the group are already colonized before the first child becomes ill. Indeed, the ill child usually acquires the bacteria from other healthy children who are carrying the organism.

Incubation Period ▸ The incubation period is from 2 days to several weeks. Most people who acquire the organism become temporarily colonized (for weeks to months) with the bacteria and never develop an invasive, symptomatic infection. The majority of the people who do develop an invasive infection do so within 1 week of exposure. However, because the exposure may be to an asymptomatic carrier rather than to an ill person, it is often impossible to identify accurately the time of exposure.

DIAGNOSIS

The diagnosis is usually made by recovering the bacteria from the cerebrospinal fluid or from the bloodstream. This is accomplished by culturing specimens obtained by performing a lumbar puncture (spinal tap) and by drawing a sample of the blood. Throat cultures are not useful for establishing a diagnosis because of the high carriage rate.

TREATMENT

Children with meningococcal infections are usually hospitalized and treated with an intravenous antibiotic.

INFECTIOUS PERIOD

The occurrence of a meningococcal infection is a marker for a high rate of colonization in the entire daycare group or preschool class. Consequently, even though the ill child's infectivity diminishes dramatically within 24 hours of the initiation of antibiotic therapy, the organism may continue to spread within the center from other healthy, colonized children.

INFECTION CONTROL

Parental Advice ▶ Prophylactic antimicrobials should be administered promptly to all children and adults in the exposed group. It is usually prudent to try to identify one knowledgeable physician to direct this effort. If each parent goes to his or her own physician, there may be several conflicting recommendations. As the goal of chemoprophylaxis is to eliminate colonization in the entire group, its effectiveness is directly related to the completeness and timeliness with which chemoprophylaxis is implemented.

Parents should realize that most children who are exposed do not become ill. However, at the first sign of an illness that is compatible with a meningococcal infection (fever and/or a petechial rash, which is one that doesn't fade in color when you apply pressure), the child should be evaluated promptly by a physician.

Vaccine ▶ The meningococcal conjugate vaccine is routinely recommended in the United States for all children older than 10 years of age and for high risk children 2 to 10 years of age. High risk infants and toddlers may be immunized beginning at 2 months of age.

Exclusion from Daycare or Preschool Attendance ▶ The child may return as soon as he or she recovers after treatment.

Recommendations for Other Children ▶ Chemoprophylaxis with rifampin or ceftriaxone is effective for eliminating colonization with the meningococcus. Rifampin or ceftriaxone should be administered to all other children who are regularly cared for in the same room. Rifampin may impart an orangish-red color to urine, tears, and other bodily fluids. Children who develop fever or other symptoms that are consistent with a meningococcal infection should be evaluated promptly by a physician.

Recommendations for Personnel ▶ Rifampin, ceftriaxone or ciprofloxacin should be administered to all personnel who are regularly in the same room (ceftriaxone may be preferred for pregnant women). Ciprofloxacin is not recommended in certain areas where strains that are resistant to the drug have emerged. Personnel in whom fever or other symptoms develop that are consistent with a meningococcal infection should be evaluated promptly by a physician.

41

MOLLUSCUM CONTAGIOSUM

Leigh B. Grossman
Vincent Iannelli

SIGNS AND SYMPTOMS

Molluscum contagiosum is an infection of the superficial skin layers that is characterized by small 2- to 5-millimeter papules that have a small central indentation on each lesion and a central core, that, if expressed, produce a typical, white exudate. The lesions of *Molluscum contagiosum* infection usually present as:

- small groups of lesions found on the face, trunk, and limbs of children;

- groups of lesions found on the abdomen, inner thighs, and genitals of sexually active adults; or

- widespread and long-standing eruptions in immunocompromised patients (e.g., AIDS, transplantation, etc.).

The lesions are benign in the healthy child, are usually painless, and the patient is otherwise asymptomatic. Children can sometimes have areas around the lesions that are red, scaling, and itchy and this is called molluscum dermatitis or molluscum eczema.

The lesions classically disappear spontaneously within 6 to 12 months. However, during that time period, some children may have as many as 50 lesions or more.

CAUSE

The *Molluscum contagiosum* virus is a DNA virus in the poxvirus family.

SPREAD AND CONTROL

Source of the Organism ► Humans.

High-Risk Populations ► The immunocompromised patient may develop widespread lesions, individual lesions that are larger than the usual molluscum lesions, and lesions that are resistant to standard therapy. Patients with allergic skin disease, as a result of the disruption of their skin integrity and their propensity to scratch, may be at greater risk of acquiring this infection and more likely to autoinoculate their skin in other regions.

Mode of Spread ► The mode of spread of *Molluscum contagiosum* is by direct human-to-human contact, indirect spread via contaminated objects such as towels, or by autoinoculation.

Incubation Period ► The incubation period has not been well studied, but it is estimated to be between 2 weeks to 6 months following exposure.

DIAGNOSIS

The diagnosis of *Molluscum contagiosum* is usually made based on the classic clinical appearance of the skin papules with their central indentation. Skin biopsy may be necessary in the immunocompromised patient to rule out other disorders. The biopsy shows the classic "molluscum bodies" which are inclusions that have a particular eosinophilic staining pattern and are only in the superficial layers of the skin or in the expressed core material from the papule. The differential diagnosis includes cryptoccocosis, basal cell carcinoma, keratoacanthoma, histoplasmosis, coccidiomycosis, and *Verruca vulgaris.* If the lesions are only in the genital region in young children, sexual abuse should be considered and the differential diagnosis would be extended to include condylomata acuminata, and vaginal syringomas. A child with molluscum in the genital region should be screened for other sexually transmitted diseases.

TREATMENT

Treatment is unnecessary in most healthy individuals because this infection is self-limited and typically disappears spontaneously over a 6- to 12-month period. If the lesions are visually noticeable, are spreading rapidly, or the child has underlying atopic dermatitis and thus is more likely to self-inoculate other places and/or there is a risk of transmission, the treatment options are:

- cryotherapy of each lesion,
- curettage of each lesion,
- laser therapy of each lesion,
- oral cimetidine, or
- topical podophyllotoxin cream, iodine, salicyclic acid, potassium hydroxide, tretinoin, cantharidin, or imiquimod.

INFECTIOUS PERIOD

Children are infectious for as long as they have visible *Molluscum contagiosum* lesions.

INFECTION CONTROL

Parental Advice ▸ All parents should recognize that *Molluscum contagiosum* is a benign skin infection and should seek medical attention for their child if he/she develops any new lesions. If their child has *Molluscum contagiosum* lesions, the lesions should be covered with clothing, if possible, or a watertight dressing to avoid transmission to other children and/or other areas of uninfected skin in their own child (autoinoculation).

Vaccine ▸ There is no available vaccine.

Exclusion from Daycare or Preschool Attendance ▶ *Molluscum contagiosum* is not harmful and should not prevent a child from attending daycare or preschool.

Recommendations for Other Children ▶ Any child with new bumps or lesions should wash their hands frequently and any new lesion should be seen by a physician.

Recommendations for Personnel ▶ All adults should make certain that, when possible, lesions are covered with clothing and/or a watertight dressing. Personnel should practice scrupulous handwashing in caring for all children.

42

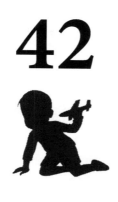

MUMPS

Gregory F. Hayden

SIGNS AND SYMPTOMS

The clinical spectrum of mumps is broad, ranging from sub-clinical infection to severe illness with involvement of many organ systems. Clinical diagnosis generally depends upon swelling of the salivary glands with prominent parotid gland enlargement. Other organ system involvement may include the brain (meningoencephalitis), the ears (usually unilateral deafness), the pancreas, the joints (arthritis), the heart (myocarditis), the thyroid gland, the kidneys (nephritis), and the liver (hepatitis). Orchitis or testicular inflammation develops in approximately 20 to 30 percent of affected postpubertal males, but only about 25 percent of such cases are bilateral, and only a small fraction of these develop progressive testicular atrophy.

CAUSE

Mumps is caused by an RNA virus. There is only one serologic type.

SPREAD AND CONTROL

Reported mumps in the United States has declined substantially since the mumps virus vaccine was licensed in 1967. Only 200 to 300 mumps cases were being reported annually until 2006 and there have been subsequent sporadic epidemics in college students and religious communities, and, most recently, in sports teams and specific states.

Source of the Organism ▸ Humans are the only natural host.

High-Risk Populations ▸ Mumps infections are uncommon in the first several months of life, but, after this age, unvaccinated children remain at high risk of developing mumps if exposed. The 2006 and 2009 outbreaks affected primarily adolescents and young adults, many of whom had previously received mumps vaccine, suggesting possible waning of vaccine-induced immunity. The risk of mumps complications, such as orchitis, meningoencephalitis, and arthritis, is higher in older patients.

Mode of Spread ▸ The virus is spread by droplets and by direct contact with respiratory secretions of an infected patient.

Incubation Period ▸ The incubation period is usually 16 to 18 days, but it can range from 12 to 25 days.

DIAGNOSIS

The clinical diagnosis of mumps can be confirmed by using viral culture or tests which detect antibodies. Polymerase chain reaction (PCR) testing has been used to detect the mumps virus. A suspected or confirmed diagnosis of mumps should be reported immediately to the local health department.

TREATMENT

No specific therapy is currently available. The selection of treatment, therefore, depends solely on the presence and severity of associated symptoms. Warm or cold compresses and analgesic therapy with acetaminophen, for example, may be used to relieve parotid gland discomfort. A soft, bland diet may be preferred. Hospitalization is recommended only for those occasional children with very severe or complicated cases requiring intensive supportive care. Children with severe central nervous system involvement, for example, may require hospitalization for bed rest, analgesic/antipyretic therapy, and carefully monitored intravenous fluid therapy.

INFECTIOUS PERIOD

Patients are most contagious from 1 to 2 days before the onset of parotid swelling until 5 days after the onset of swelling. Virus has been isolated from saliva up to 7 days before the onset of parotid swelling until as long as 9 days after onset.

INFECTION CONTROL

Parental Advice ► Parents should be advised that a suspected (or confirmed) case of mumps has occurred in a child at the center. They should be advised that the risk to their child is minimal so long as the child has already received mumps vaccine. Parents of unimmunized children should be advised to seek medical advice immediately concerning the prompt vaccination of children older than 1 year of age. Parents should also be urged to verify their own immunity status as well as the immunization status of any older children in the family, especially adolescents, who do not attend the center, and to seek vaccination as appropriate.

Vaccine ► Live, attenuated mumps virus vaccine should be given routinely to children after the first birthday and is usually administered at 12 to 15 months of age as a part of the combined measles-mumps-rubella (MMR) vaccine or the combined measles-mumps-rubella-varicella (MMRV vaccine). The cornerstone of mumps prevention in daycare centers and preschools should be the vigilant insistence that all children 15 months or older have received the mumps vaccine as a prerequisite for attending the center. A single dose of vaccine confers long-lasting mumps immunity and the second recommended dose at 4 to 6 years of age maximizes the effectiveness and provides an added safeguard against primary vaccine failures.

Precautions and contraindications to live mumps vaccination include altered immunity, anaphylactic allergy to neomycin or gelatin, severe febrile illness, pregnancy, and recent receipt of an immune globulin preparation or blood products. Persons with allergy to eggs should receive mumps vaccine only with caution, but most children with egg hypersensitivity can be safely immunized with the MMR vaccine. MMR vaccine is recommended for children infected with the human immunodeficiency virus if they are not in severely immunocompromised condition.

Exclusion from Daycare or Preschool Attendance ▶ Because the period of maximum communicability extends until 5 days after the onset of parotid swelling, infected children should be excluded for this interval. By this time, the parotid swelling should have subsided, and any other manifestations of mumps should have resolved. As patients are often contagious before the onset of parotid swelling, however, and because inapparent infections can be communicable, attempts to control spread by means of isolation are commonly ineffective.

Recommendations for Other Children ▶ The first step is to verify that other children attending the center have already been immunized against mumps in accordance with established center policy. Children with documented previous immunization against mumps are highly unlikely to develop illness and may continue to attend the center. In the unlikely occurrence of an outbreak involving young children, a second dose of mumps vaccine could be considered for children 1 to 4 years old (at a minimum interval of 28 days between doses), recognizing that the vaccine may not be effective in preventing already incubating mumps infection.

The management of unvaccinated children is somewhat more complex. It is not known whether the administration of mumps vaccine after exposure can prevent or modify illness. Adverse reactions to this vaccine are uncommon, however, and vaccination after exposure is not known to increase the severity of incubating mumps. If an exposed child is not already incubating infection, mumps vaccination should protect the child against subsequent exposures to mumps. Vaccination can, therefore, be recommended for unimmunized children at least 12 months of age, especially if they have been exposed for no more than a few days. Parents must understand, however, that the vaccine may not block the progression of already incubating mumps, so that they will not wrongly blame the vaccine for mumps illness that develops after vaccination.

For children younger than 1 year of age, vaccination is a less attractive option because it is not as effective in creating a protective immune response in this age group. Standard immunoglobulin is ineffective in protecting against mumps infection. These infants could be excluded from the center during the period when they might be expected to become ill and contagious themselves. Because patients may be contagious up to 7 days before the onset of parotid swelling and because the incubation period may vary from 12 to 25 days, this policy would require exclusion of infants from the daycare center or preschool for 3 weeks or longer. As mumps is usually not severe in young infants, simple observation seems reasonable if coupled with careful documentation of immunization among those 12 months of age or older. If additional cases of mumps were to occur among younger infants, however, a strict exclusionary policy could then be enforced.

Recommendations for Personnel ► Ideally, all staff members should provide a documented history of adequate mumps immunization, a physician-documented diagnosis of previous infection, or serologic evidence of immunity at the time of employment. Adequate immunization has been defined as 1 dose of mumps vaccine for adults not at high risk of exposure, and 2 doses for those at high risk of exposure (such as health care workers, international travelers, and students at post–high school educational institutions). As relatively few cases of mumps are currently reported in young children, most daycare center and preschool staff are at low risk for mumps exposure. If mumps were to become reported more commonly in young children, however, the risk of mumps exposures among staff workers would increase, and a second dose of mumps vaccine could be considered. Birth before 1957 is generally considered presumptive evidence of immunity to mumps because most individuals born before 1957 will have contracted mumps illness as a child and developed natural immunity. If mumps were to become more common in young children, however, unvaccinated staff members born before 1957 who do not have either a history of physician-diagnosed mumps or laboratory evidence of mumps immunity could consider receiving one dose of mumps vaccine.

Strict adherence to such a policy reduces or eliminates the disruption that can arise among personnel when mumps is diagnosed in a child attending the center. If appropriate preparations have not been made before such a case occurs, the first step is to determine whether any center personnel are likely to be susceptible to mumps using blood tests to document immunity on historical information. A history of having received 2 doses of mumps vaccine previously is highly, but not perfectly, predictive of mumps immunity. A history of physician-diagnosed mumps illness is also highly predictive of mumps immunity. In contrast, a negative history of mumps illness is poorly predictive of mumps susceptibility. Most adults with such negative histories are immune to mumps on the basis of previous, unrecognized infection. Most persons born before 1957 are immune, but if such persons lack a history of physician-diagnosed mumps or laboratory evidence of mumps immunity, they may consider receiving a single dose of mumps vaccine for added protection. Younger adults with a negative history of mumps immunization or illness are at somewhat greater risk of infection and can consider immunization after the exposure, recognizing that the vaccine may not be effective in preventing incubating mumps infection.

43

MYCOPLASMA PNEUMONIAE

(Pneumonia)

Ronald B. Turner

SIGNS AND SYMPTOMS

Mycoplasma pneumoniae infection may result in symptoms at any level of the respiratory tract. Pneumonia is the most commonly recognized manifestation of infection and is characterized by prominent cough and fever. Other respiratory syndromes associated with mycoplasma infection are pharyngitis (sore throat) and bronchiolitis. Most preschool children infected with mycoplasma are asymptomatic.

M. pneumoniae has rarely been associated with a variety of non-respiratory illnesses. Joint and heart involvement and a variety of neurologic syndromes have been reported in patients infected with *M. pneumoniae*. These manifestations of infection have generally been reported in patients older than those who would be seen in a daycare setting.

CAUSE

Mycoplasmas are free-living organisms that can be cultured.

SPREAD AND CONTROL

Source of the Organism ▶ Infected humans are the only known source of infection.

High-Risk Populations ▶ No populations have been identified that are at high risk for acquisition of infection. Infection of children with sickle cell disease has been associated with more severe respiratory disease.

Mode of Spread ▶ The mechanism of transmission is not known with certainty but is thought to be person-to-person spread by large-particle aerosols. Small-particle aerosols may rarely play a role in transmission of infection.

Incubation Period ▶ The incubation period for mycoplasma infection is 2 to 3 weeks.

DIAGNOSIS

Culture of *M. pneumoniae* is relatively easily accomplished by experienced personnel. The organism grows slowly, however, so culture is generally not useful in the clinical setting. Serology (test for antibodies) has been the cornerstone of the diagnosis of *M. pneumoniae* infections. Diagnostic testing by polymerase chain reaction (PCR) is available.

TREATMENT

Erythromycin is the usual treatment for mycoplasma infections in children. Azithromycin is also effective against mycoplasma. Hospitalization is usually not necessary.

INFECTIOUS PERIOD

The period of infectivity is not known; however, infected individuals should be considered capable of transmitting infection for the duration of the cough.

INFECTION CONTROL

Parental Advice ► Mycoplasma infections spread very slowly and have not been associated with outbreaks in the daycare or preschool setting. No special precautions are indicated.

Vaccine ► None available.

Exclusion from Daycare or Preschool Attendance ► Exclusion from daycare or preschool settings is not necessary for children infected with mycoplasma.

Recommendations for Other Children ► No special precautions are indicated.

Recommendations for Personnel ► No special precautions are indicated.

44

NECATOR AMERICANUS

(Hookworm)

Jonathan P. Moorman

SIGNS AND SYMPTOMS

The initial manifestation of an infection with *Necator americanus* may consist of itching and burning ("ground itch"), followed by the development of a rash that looks like small bumps or vesicles at the site where the larvae penetrate the skin. Although many infected individuals never have symptoms, heavy infections can be associated with the development of gastrointestinal symptoms, including abdominal pain, anorexia, diarrhea, and weight loss. The most debilitating effect of hookworm infections is chronic intestinal blood loss resulting in the development of iron-deficiency anemia. The severity of the anemia is variable, depending on the worm burden and dietary iron intake. The average daily loss of blood for this worm is less significant than the loss that occurs with *Ancylostoma duodenale* hookworm infections. It may be associated with pallor, decreased energy, shortness of breath, palpitations, increase in heart size, and impaired growth. The blood, heart, and nutritional effects of hookworm infections contribute significantly to illness in child and adult populations worldwide.

CAUSE

N. americanus is one of the two most common hookworms found in humans. Along with *A. duodenale*, it affects one quarter of the world's population. Humans acquire the infection through the skin by coming into contact with infective larvae present in contaminated soil. The larvae penetrate the skin, migrate through the blood to the lungs, pass through the alveolar walls, and ascend the trachea. They are then swallowed and move to the small intestine where they attach to the small bowel and jejunal mucosa and mature into adults. After mating, the female worms lay eggs, discharging thousands per day in the feces. Under favorable environmental soil conditions, the eggs in the soil will hatch and larvae will develop into infective forms. This process generally requires 5 to 10 days in the soil, only after which they become infective for humans.

SPREAD AND CONTROL

Source of the Organism ▸ Hookworms continue to be endemic in a number of tropical and subtropical areas. *N. americanus* is the prevailing species in parts of the southern United States, Central and South America, the Caribbean, central and southern Africa, and southern Asia. Hookworm has remained endemic in areas where fecal pollution and environmental conditions favoring the development of hookworm eggs are present. The infective larvae are found in soil contaminated with human feces, and transmission is generally the result of direct contact with the soil, often through bare feet. Although transmission of *A. duodenale* occurs through food and possibly breast milk, this does not appear to occur with *N. americanus*.

High-Risk Populations ▸ Individuals who have direct contact with fecally contaminated soil in hookworm-endemic areas will be at risk of acquiring the infection. Because children are more likely to go barefoot and to play in dirt, they are also more likely to acquire hookworm infections. However, as the larvae are not infective unless they undergo development in soil, direct person-to-person spread of hookworm does not appear to occur. Therefore, institutional or childcare settings should not increase a child's risk of infection.

Mode of Spread ▶ Transmission occurs via the skin when there is contact with soil containing infective hookworm larvae. Larvae require 5 to 10 minutes of contact for penetration.

Incubation Period ▶ The time interval between the acquisition of *N. americanus* and the passage of eggs in the feces ranges from approximately 40 to 60 days. Considerable variability has also been observed in the time between exposure and development of symptoms; some individuals develop gastrointestinal symptoms 20 to 45 days following an acute infection.

DIAGNOSIS

The diagnosis is established by identifying the characteristic hookworm eggs in feces; *N. americanus* eggs cannot be distinguished from those of *A. duodenale*. Most moderate to severe hookworm infections will be detected by direct microscopic examination of a fecal smear. However, the detection of light infections may require the use of concentration techniques.

TREATMENT

In countries where hookworm infections are endemic and re-infection is common, light infections are often not treated. In this country, hookworm infections are generally treated with either mebendazole, albendazole, or pyrantel pamoate. Although pyrantel pamoate and albendazole are recommended drugs, the U.S. Food and Drug Administration considers them investigational for this condition. These regimens appear to be well tolerated, but experience with them in children less than 2 years of age is limited, and therefore, the decision to treat a child in this age group should be made on an individual basis after determining the potential risks and benefits of therapy. A repeat stool examination should be performed 1 to 2 weeks following therapy, and retreatment should be undertaken if hookworm infection is persistent. In addition to the use of anti-parasitic agents, iron supplementation should be provided to individuals with significant anemia.

INFECTIOUS PERIOD

If untreated, hookworm infections, in particular those caused by *N. americanus*, may persist for many years. Because egg production tends to decrease over time, individuals may become somewhat less infectious.

INFECTION CONTROL

Parental Advice ▶ Parents should be told that the risk of person-to-person transmission is minimal. If the attendee appears to have acquired the infection locally, the need for sanitary disposal of feces and the potential for spread through contaminated soil should be reviewed with all of the parents.

Vaccine ▶ None available, although several candidates are currently being studied.

Exclusion from Daycare or Preschool Attendance ▶ Children with hookworm infections do not need to be isolated. Because human-to-human transmission does not occur and the eggs passed in feces are not infectious, an infected child does not need to be kept out of any childcare setting.

Recommendations for Other Children ▶ Other children will acquire hookworm only if they come into contact with soil containing infective larvae. Unlike the situation with many other gastrointestinal pathogens, children do not become infected if they inadvertently ingest fecal material contaminated with hookworm eggs. Therefore, no additional precautions need to be undertaken for children in a center when one child is found to have hookworm infection.

Recommendations for Personnel ▶ Personnel should be instructed to maintain techniques that decrease fecal–oral transmission of pathogens, including good handwashing and appropriate disposal of fecal material. Obviously, no child should be allowed to defecate in the playground areas where fecal contamination of the soil may be a problem, and children should not be allowed to go barefoot or play in the soil.

45

PAPILLOMAVIRUSES

(Warts)

David A. Whiting

SIGNS AND SYMPTOMS

Warts are unusual in infancy and early childhood and have a peak incidence at 12 to 16 years of age. Warts are usually small skin and mucous membrane tumors and are caused by a DNA virus known as the human papillomavirus (HPV).

Common warts (Verruca vulgaris): These occur as firm papules with a rough, horny surface that range in size from 1 to 12 millimeters in diameter and are usually separate lesions, but may merge to become one large wart. They often contain black specks on the surface from thrombosed capillaries. They can occur anywhere on the body but are seen most commonly on the backs of the hands and fingers and on the knees. Sixty-five percent disappear spontaneously within 2 years.

Plane warts (Verruca plana): These are multiple, small, tan or flesh-colored, flattened, round, or polygonal lesions 1 to 5 millimeters in diameter and are found mostly on the face, backs of the hands, and shins.

Plantar warts (Verruca plantaris): These are inverted, flattened, circumscribed horny papules of the soles often containing black specks from thrombosed capillaries. Plantar warts may be single, multiple, or mosaic. They are rare in the pre-school-aged child.

Venereal warts (Condylomata acuminata): These manifest as multiple pointed bumps, single or confluent, on or around the genitalia and the anus. In children, the possibility of child abuse should always be considered in cases of venereal warts.

CAUSE

Human papillomaviruses are small, double-stranded DNA viruses. More than 130 types of HPV have now been identified and there are common viral types associated with different warts.

Common warts (Verruca vulgaris): HPV 2, 4, 29, 57.

Plane warts (Verruca plana): HPV 3, 10.

Plantar warts (Verruca plantaris): HPV 1, 2, 4, 10.

Venereal warts (Condylomata acuminata): HPV 6, 11, 42, 54

SPREAD AND CONTROL

Source of the Organism ► Other humans.

High-Risk Populations ► Schoolchildren 12 to 16 years of age or immunosuppressed individuals are at high risk. Abused children may have genital warts.

Mode of Spread ► Warts are spread by direct contact with an infected individual, by indirect contact through contamination of objects and immediate environment, and by self-inocula-tion from another site.

Incubation Period ► One to 20 months, with an average of 4 months.

DIAGNOSIS

The clinical appearance is usually diagnostic, and the presence of warts may be confirmed by demonstrating black dots in them after paring down the horny surfaces. A biopsy is some-times diagnostic. HPV testing can be confirmatory.

TREATMENT

Therapy is local and is done on an outpatient basis. Hospital admission is not required unless it is for very extensive vene-real warts.

There is no specific antiviral therapy, although an injection into the lesion of alpha-2b interferon has been used success-fully in some cases, and topically applied imiquimod cream is indicated for genital warts.

Common warts: Light electrodesiccation and curettage, cryo-surgery, keratolytics, monochloroacetic acid or bichloracetic acid, laser surgery.

Plane warts: Cryosurgery, monochloroacetic acid or bichloracetic acid, light electrodesiccation and curettage, topical tretinoin and imiquimod cream.

Plantar warts: Keratolytics, light electrodesiccation and curettage, formalin soaks, laser surgery. Cryosurgery is painful when treating the soles of the feet.

Venereal warts: Podophyllin (25 percent) in compound tincture of benzoin or podophyllotoxin, imiquimod cream, monochloroacetic acid or bichloracetic acid, cryosurgery, light electrodesiccation and curettage, laser surgery.

Note that a wait-and-see attitude is advisable in children, as many warts disappear spontaneously and wart treatment is often destructive and painful and liable to cause scars. The least destructive therapy possible is always advisable.

INFECTIOUS PERIOD

How long the infectious period will last is uncertain, but it may last as long as the lesion is actually present, which can be months or years.

INFECTION CONTROL

Parental Advice ▸ Wait and see if warts develop, and treat if necessary.

Vaccine ▸ Two vaccines have been FDA approved for the prevention of HPV infection and are recommended for administration prior to the initiation of sexual activity. Both contain HPV strains 16 and 18, which cause 70 percent of the cervical cancer cases in the United States, and one also contains HPV strains 6 and 11, which commonly cause genital warts.

Exclusion from Daycare or Preschool Attendance ▸ Isolation is unnecessary, although it is advisable to cover the warts, if practical.

Recommendations for Other Children ▸ Wait and see if warts develop, and treat if necessary.

Recommendations for Personnel ▸ Wait and see if warts develop, and treat if necessary.

46

PARAINFLUENZA VIRUS

Scott A. Halperin

SIGNS AND SYMPTOMS

Parainfluenza virus causes both upper and lower respiratory tract disease in children. Upper respiratory infection with fever is the most common manifestation of parainfluenza virus infection and is indistinguishable from the common cold caused by other viruses. The disease is characterized by runny nose, cough, and sore throat and may be associated with a low-grade fever.

Parainfluenza virus is the most common infectious agent causing croup, which is characterized by hoarseness, a barking cough, and inspiratory stridor. Parainfluenza viruses also are important causes of bronchiolitis, bronchitis, and pneumonia. Outbreaks of croup caused by parainfluenza virus often occur each fall, although sporadic infection occurs throughout the year. Reinfections with parainfluenza virus occur but are usually mild.

CAUSE

Parainfluenza viruses are enveloped RNA viruses that are similar to the influenza virus. There are four specific types that cause disease in humans. Parainfluenza virus types 1 and 2 are the most common causes of croup, while parainfluenza virus type 3 is an important cause of pneumonia and bronchiolitis. Types 1, 2, and 3 also are associated with symptoms of the common cold. Parainfluenza virus type 4 causes very mild disease of the upper respiratory tract.

SPREAD AND CONTROL

Source of the Organism ► Parainfluenza virus is spread from person to person or found in infected respiratory secretions. Although parainfluenza-like viruses exist in animals, these do not cause infection or disease in humans.

High-Risk Populations ► Infants and young children are susceptible to parainfluenza viruses, and almost all children will have been infected with all four types by the age of 6 years. The severity of the illness depends on the parainfluenza virus type, the age of the child, and whether it is a primary infection or a reinfection. Severe prolonged infection can occur in children who have impaired immune function

Mode of Spread ► Parainfluenza viruses are spread from person to person by direct contact or by large droplets and contaminated nasopharyngeal secretions.

Incubation Period ► Two to 4 days.

DIAGNOSIS

Specific virologic diagnosis of parainfluenza virus infection is not routinely necessary because treatment is nonspecific and symptomatic. Because of the epidemic nature of certain parainfluenza virus infections, a diagnosis can occasionally be deduced by using knowledge of the predominant viral infection in a community at that time. When indicated, virologic diagnosis of parainfluenza virus infection can be established by isolating the virus in tissue culture. The diagnosis can also be made (a) by detection of the virus in infected secretions by using direct or indirect immunofluorescent techniques, (b) by antigen detection methods, or (c) by nucleic acid detection such as polymerase chain reaction (PCR). Specific diagnosis of parainfluenza virus infections is becoming more frequent as

PCR assays are available that detect a range of different respiratory pathogens from a single specimen.

TREATMENT

No specific antiviral therapy is yet available for parainfluenza virus infection. Most infections due to parainfluenza virus are self-limited; however, parainfluenza virus infections of the lower respiratory tract may be severe and require hospitalization for supportive care. Oxygen, epinephrine, and oral, intravenous or intramuscular, and aerosolized steroid therapy are effective in the management of some patients with croup.

INFECTIOUS PERIOD

Parainfluenza viruses may be shed for 4 to 21 days, depending on the type.

INFECTION CONTROL

Parental Advice ▶ No specific precautions are indicated.

Vaccine ▶ No vaccine is currently available but several candidate vaccines are being studied.

Exclusion from Daycare or Preschool Attendance ▶ Exclusion from daycare or preschool settings is not necessary for children infected with parainfluenza virus.

Recommendations for Other Children ▶ No specific precautions are indicated.

Recommendations for Personnel ▶ No specific precautions are indicated.

47

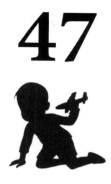

PARVOVIRUS B19

(Fifth Disease, Erythema Infectiosum)

William C. Koch

SIGNS AND SYMPTOMS

The most common manifestation of infection with the human parvovirus B19 is a benign rash illness of childhood called erythema infectiosum (EI) or "Fifth Disease." EI occurs most often in school-aged children, with a peak season from late winter to early spring. The illness begins with an early phase of mild fever and nonspecific symptoms of headache, malaise, and myalgia. This phase lasts only a few days and is followed by the eruption of the characteristic rash. This begins as an intensely red symmetric facial rash, giving the child a "slapped-cheek" appearance. It then spreads to the trunk and the extremities as an erythematous, raised rash. As the rash progresses, there is central clearing that gives it a reticular or lacy character, especially on the arms and legs. The palms and soles are usually spared. When the rash appears, the child has almost always begun to feel better, and fever, if present, resolves. The rash may persist for weeks and may recur in response to various stimuli such as exposure to sunlight, a warm bath, or exercise.

B19 also causes more serious illnesses in other groups of individuals. These include a syndrome of acute, self-limited arthropathy in adults; transient bone marrow suppression with low blood counts in individuals with chronic hemolytic anemia such as sickle cell anemia or hereditary spherocytosis; fetal hydrops and stillbirth in pregnant women; and chronic anemia in adults and children with impaired immunity. Asymptomatic infections occur commonly, and atypical rashes have been reported with this infection, including an unusual dermatologic syndrome called the papular-purpuric "gloves and socks" syndrome, characterized by fever, swelling, and a petechial rash over the hands and feet. There is no evidence that parvovirus B19 causes congenital anomalies.

CAUSE

Parvovirus B19 is a small DNA virus. It is one of the smallest DNA-containing viruses known to infect mammalian cells. There is only one serotype of parvovirus B19.

SPREAD AND CONTROL

Source of the Organism ▶ The virus is contracted from infected individuals during the period of time in their illness when they have the virus in their blood. Virus can be detected in respiratory secretions at this time, suggesting that these secretions are involved in transmission. For patients with EI, this occurs during the early phase, prior to the onset of the rash. In patients with parvovirus B19-induced aplastic crisis or chronic anemia, the time period when the virus is in the bloodstream occurs at clinical presentation and is of much greater intensity.

High-Risk Populations ▶ There are no underlying conditions that predispose to acquisition of parvovirus B19 infection. Although the infection occurs most commonly in school-aged children, it can be spread to their younger siblings through household contact and is thus subsequently introduced into the daycare or preschool setting. There are certain groups who are at risk for more serious consequences if they acquire a parvovirus B19 infection, and these include children with conditions of chronic hemolysis (e.g., sickle cell disease), immunocompromised patients (including human immunodeficiency virus [HIV] infection), and pregnant women.

Mode of Spread ▸ The virus is spread by close contact, presumably through respiratory secretions. The secondary attack rate for susceptible household contacts is about 30 to 50 percent. In school outbreaks, the secondary attack rate has varied from 10 to 60 percent. Potential mechanisms of transmission include direct personal contact, large-particle and small-particle droplets, and fomites (shared objects and surfaces such as toys, doorknobs, etc.). Transmission by blood or blood products is also possible.

Incubation Period ▸ The incubation period for EI is reported to range from 4 to 14 days on average, with the longest reported incubation time being 28 days. However, results of experimental parvovirus B19 infection in adults suggest an incubation period of 17 to 18 days based on time to onset of the rash. The incubation period for the parvovirus B19-related aplastic crisis is generally shorter as it coincides with the onset of viremia, usually 6 to 8 days after exposure.

DIAGNOSIS

EI is usually diagnosed clinically by documenting the classic prodrome, or early phase of the illness, followed by the classic rash. It can be confirmed by serologic tests for parvovirus B19 antibodies. The most reliable single test for acute infection is detection of anti-B19 immunoglobulin M (IgM). This is detectable by 8 to 10 days after infection and persists for 2 to 3 months. Infection can also be diagnosed by seroconversion from negative to positive on a test for anti-B19 immunoglobulin G (IgG) antibody. IgG is detectable a few days after IgM and persists for life. These serologic tests are available at commercial laboratories and some state health departments. In immunocompromised patients, specific antibody production may be impaired, so diagnosis usually requires detection of viral DNA by nucleic acid hybridization or polymerase chain reaction (PCR) tests.

TREATMENT

Children with EI require no therapy, as the great majority will recover without incident. Children with aplastic crisis will usually require hospitalization for supportive care with oxygen and transfusions until their hematocrit and hemoglobin return to baseline. There is no antiviral therapy available. Although the use of commercial preparations of immune globulin have been reported to ameliorate parvovirus B19 infections in immunocompromised children, their use as either treatment or post-exposure prophylaxis in pregnant caretakers cannot be recommended until further studies are performed.

INFECTIOUS PERIOD

Children with EI are infectious during the early phase of their illness when the virus is detectable in their respiratory secretions, a period of 1 to 6 days. This phase may go unnoticed but usually occurs about 7 to 10 days prior to the onset of the rash. The appearance of the rash coincides with production of virus-specific antibodies and once the rash develops the child is no longer infectious.

INFECTION CONTROL

Parental Advice ▸ Once an outbreak of EI has been identified in a center, parents of children in attendance should be informed of the risk for transmission of the virus both in the center and from susceptible contacts at home. They should be made aware of the generally benign nature of the illness and those underlying conditions that are considered higher risk. Those families who desire more information about parvovirus B19 infections should be referred to their health care provider or local health officials.

Vaccine ▸ None available.

Exclusion from Daycare or Preschool Attendance ▸ Children with EI do not need to be excluded from daycare, as they are unlikely to be infectious after the rash appears and the clinical diagnosis is made. Children with aplastic crisis are infectious at presentation with fever and anemia, and they remain infectious for a longer period of time. Such children will most likely be hospitalized until their hematologic status is stable. They should be isolated for at least 1 week after presentation and should not return to the daycare or preschool setting until after this time.

Recommendations for Other Children ► Once an outbreak of EI has been identified in a daycare center or preschool, parents of children at risk for more serious complications as a result of parvovirus B19 infection (chronic hemolytic conditions, immunocompromised, etc.) should be notified. They may wish to consult their pediatricians for individual advice. A general policy of exclusion is not recommended.

Recommendations for Personnel ► There are no studies documenting the effectiveness of handwashing or decontamination of toys and environmental surfaces in preventing the transmission of parvovirus B19; however, handwashing and careful control of respiratory secretions are recommended.

When an outbreak of EI is identified in a center, there is some risk that the adult personnel will become infected. This is primarily of concern for those who are pregnant. Approximately 50 percent of adults will already be seropositive and, therefore, immune to infection. If a pregnant woman becomes infected, the risk of an adverse outcome (e.g., fetal loss) caused by parvovirus B19 is low, with risk estimates ranging from 1.6 to 6 percent in large studies. Infection occurring in the first half of pregnancy appears to be associated with the highest risk. Personnel who are pregnant should be aware of ways to minimize exposure by proper handwashing, avoidance of shared utensils, etc. If available, serologic testing for the presence of anti-B19 IgG could be of benefit by identifying those women who are already immune and thus not at risk of being infected. Individuals who desire more information on the risks and management of parvovirus B19 exposure should contact their health care provider. Again, a routine policy of exclusion of pregnant caretakers is not recommended.

48

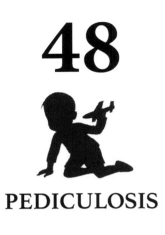

PEDICULOSIS

(Lice)

David A. Whiting

SIGNS AND SYMPTOMS

The characteristic feature of all types of lice infestation (pediculosis) is itching. Intense itching, usually worse at night, leads to scratch marks, thickened skin, pigmentation, secondary infection, and swollen lymph nodes. The actual louse bites are relatively painless and cause small, red dots. These may develop into bumps over hours or days or, in a sensitized individual, may cause immediate swelling similar to hives. The nit or egg case of the developing louse is attached firmly to human hair or threads of clothing and is usually somewhat translucent in appearance. It is often easier to find the nit than the actual louse.

Head lice: Itching is most severe around the back and sides of the scalp. Nits can be found attached to scalp hair in those areas. Scratch marks with secondary infection and lymphadenopathy is common, and foul matted hair can result. Common bacteria causing secondary infection include *Staphylococcus aureus* and group A *Streptococcus pyogenes*.

Body lice: Body lice can only survive in conditions of poor hygiene and are therefore found in homeless or displaced persons who are unable to maintain any reasonable standard of personal cleanliness. The lice live in clothing and lay eggs on the inner seams of clothes and occasionally on body hairs. Pinpoint red dots, bumps, hive-like lesions, scratches, secondary infection, and, perhaps, pigmentation can occur all over the body. Note that body lice can carry other diseases such as epidemic or louseborne typhus (caused by *Rickettsia prowazekii*), trench fever (caused by *Rochalimaea* [*Rickettsia quintana*]), and European or louseborne relapsing fever (caused by *Borrelia recurrentis*). Body lice are human-to-human carriers of murine typhus or are vectors of endemic or fleaborne typhus caused by *Rickettsia typhi* (*mooseri*).

Pubic lice: Pubic or crab lice affect not only the pubic hair but also the adjacent hair on the thighs, abdomen, chest, breasts, and axillae and sometimes the hair on the eyebrows, eyelashes, or scalp. Intense irritation with scratch marks and eczematization occurs. Occasionally, blue-gray dots, the so-called maculae ceruleae, are found on the lower abdomen and upper thighs.

CAUSE

Sucking lice of the order Anoplura are flattened, wingless insects, and two species of these are human parasites. The first is *Pediculus humanus*, a louse 3- to 4-millimeters long that exists in humans in two distinct populations, namely, *Pediculus humanus capitis*, affecting the scalp, and *Pediculus humanus corporis*, affecting the body. The other species is *Phthirus pubis* or the crab louse, which is 2 to 3 millimeters in length and is adapted for clinging onto body hairs.

SPREAD AND CONTROL

Source of the Organism ▶ Human body.

High-Risk Populations ▶

Head lice: The greatest prevalence of head lice is usually seen in children between the ages of 3 and 10 years with equal sex incidence. More females are affected in the teens and in adult life. Head lice can affect all levels of society and all ethnic groups except for low levels of infestation in the African-

American population. Inadequate washing and grooming as seen in individuals with mental disabilities or in those with elaborate hairstyles can lead to higher populations of head lice.

Body lice: Body lice are confined to economically deprived persons who do not have a fixed home and have no means of achieving personal cleanliness. The term "vagabond's disease" is self-explanatory here. Chronically ill individuals or persons with mental disabilities who are unable to look after themselves also may be infested by body lice, and children living in that environment may become infested.

Pubic lice: Children are not usually affected by this sexually transmitted disease, but the presence of crab lice or nits in eyelashes or scalp hair in children does indicate the possibility of sexual abuse.

Mode of Spread ► Direct spread is frequent, but lice can survive for at least a week off the human body, so indirect spread can occur.

Head lice: The most common method of spread is head-to-head contact, especially in crowded sleeping quarters. Head lice can also be spread by infested headgear, towels, hairbrushes, combs, pillows, bedding, and earphones.

Body lice: Body lice are spread by person-to-person contact or contact with infested clothing or bedding.

Pubic lice: Crab lice are spread by person-to-person contact and sometimes by infested towels and bedding.

Incubation Period ► The incubation period from egg laying to the emerging adult louse is 17 to 25 days for head and body lice and 22 to 27 days for pubic lice.

DIAGNOSIS

The diagnosis is established by the identification of live lice or nits on hairs or clothing, which show pale blue fluorescence on examination using a Wood's light, or the identification of actual lice on skin, hair, or clothing. Supporting the diagnosis is a clinical picture of intense itching, scratch marks, secondary infection, and lymphadenopathy.

TREATMENT

Outpatient therapy is adequate.

Head lice: The treatment of choice, after shampooing and rinsing the hair, is to work 1 percent permethrin creme rinse into the hair and scalp, leave for 10 minutes, and then rinse it out with clear water. An alternative but less effective therapy is to apply 1 to 2 ounces of 1 percent lindane shampoo to the dry hair and work it in thoroughly, then add small quantities of water until a lather forms, and leave it in place for 4 minutes, and then rinse thoroughly and dry briskly. An effective ovicidal treatment available in various countries is 0.5 percent malathion lotion applied to the scalp once for 8 to 12 hours. One method of nit removal is a creme rinse containing 8 percent formic acid, followed by the use of a metal nit comb. A nit comb alone can also be effective. Increasing numbers of patients who are infested with lice that are resistant to permethrin are being reported. There are anecdotal reports of successful therapy for head lice with a single oral dose of ivermectin (an antihelmintic). These treatments can be repeated weekly if necessary.

Body lice: Current treatment is to sterilize clothing and bedding and to apply 1 percent lindane lotion from head to toe for 8 to 10 hours or for 6 to 8 hours in small children. A better alternative is to apply 5 percent permethrin topical cream.

Pubic lice: One method of treatment is 1 percent lindane lotion from neck to toes for 8 to 12 hours. Alternatively, 5 percent lindane shampoo can be used on the affected hair-bearing areas in the same manner as it is on the scalp, or, preferably, 1 percent permethrin creme rinse or 0.5 percent malathion can be applied.

Floors, play areas, and furniture should be vacuumed thoroughly for affected hairs. Mattresses and furniture can be sprayed with synergized pyrethrins or synthetic pyrethroids. All clothing, bedding, and headgear should be disinfected by machine washing and machine drying or dry cleaning. Clothing can also be bagged and sealed in tight plastic bags for 2 weeks. Combs and brushes should be soaked in 2 percent Lysol for 1 to 2 hours or boiled in water for 10 minutes. Combs, brushes, grooming aids, towels, sponges, and facecloths should not be shared. Any secondary infection should be treated with appropriate compresses and antibiotics.

INFECTIOUS PERIOD

The child is infectious as long as live lice or viable ova (nits) are present on the child.

INFECTION CONTROL

Parental Advice ▸ All domestic contacts should be checked for symptoms or signs and treated as necessary.

Vaccine ▸ None available.

Exclusion from Daycare or Preschool Attendance ▸ When lice have been detected and effective treatment provided, no exclusion is required.

Recommendations for Other Children ▸ Examine unaffected children for results of itching, such as scratch marks, infections, and lymphadenopathy, examine with Wood's lamp for nits, and examine for lice. If any symptoms or signs of lice are found or develop, treatment is indicated.

Recommendations for Personnel ▸ Check personnel for itching, scratch marks, infections, lymphadenopathy, nits, and lice. If any symptoms or signs develop, treatment is indicated.

49

PERTUSSIS

(Whooping Cough)

Vincent Iannelli

SIGNS AND SYMPTOMS

Pertussis evolves in three clinical stages: catarrhal (runny nose), paroxysmal (repetitive coughing), and convalescent (improving). The catarrhal stage is manifested by runny nose, nasal congestion, sneezing, mild sore throat, low-grade fever, and a mild cough. This stage lasts 1 to 2 weeks and can mimic the common cold. The paroxysmal stage follows and is manifested by more violent, protracted bouts of coughing and severe paroxysms that can last up to several minutes and which may be followed by vomiting. Gasping musical inspirations, "the whoop," often occur after these paroxysms in older infants and preschool children, but they may be absent in infants less than 6 months of age and in older children and adults. This stage lasts from 1 to 4 weeks but can last as long as 10 weeks. The convalescent stage begins when cough paroxysms cease while chronic cough continues. It usually lasts 2 to 3 weeks, with slowly decreasing frequency and severity of cough. Rarely, this stage may persist for months.

Of special note, newborns and younger infants with pertussis might have atypical symptoms. They might have a shorter catarrhal stage, during which they are at risk for periods of not breathing (apnea) and sudden death, and a longer convalescent stage.

Also, children with pertussis usually don't have high fever, conjunctivitis, wheezing, skin rashes, or tachypnea, which can help distinguish pertussis from many other childhood respiratory tract infections.

CAUSE

Pertussis, or "whooping cough," is caused by the *Bordetella pertussis* bacteria, first discovered by Jules Bordet in 1906. There are many other bacteria and viral causes of chronic cough though, such as *Bordetella parapertussis, Mycoplasma pneumoniae, Chlamydia trachomatis*, adenovirus, and respiratory syncytial virus (RSV).

SPREAD AND CONTROL

Pertussis is one of the most highly contagious diseases of humans. Attack rates approach 100 percent in close contacts who are not immune. The distribution of the disease is worldwide. It is a leading cause of sickness and death in children in developing countries where immunization against pertussis is not widely practiced.

Source of the Organism ► Humans are the only natural reservoir of *B. pertussis* organisms. Although it was once thought that there wasn't a healthy carrier state in humans for pertussis, polymerase chain reaction (PCR) testing has sometimes found a transient carrier state in some children and adults.

High-Risk Populations ► In the United States, the epidemiology of pertussis has changed dramatically over the past two decades, with the annual number of new cases of pertussis gradually increasing since 1981. Prior to 2000, the majority of pertussis cases were in infants less than 1 year of age, but since 2000 the majority of cases have been found in adolescents aged 10 to 19 years. Between 1994 and 2004 a thousand percent increase was seen in the reported incidence of pertussis in the 10- to 19-year age group. Before the routine use of pertussis vaccines in the 1940s, pertussis cases were found mainly in children between 1 and 5 years of age.

Adolescents and adults are the major reservoir of pertussis and a significant source of infection for infants and children. Adolescents and adults should be considered susceptible to pertussis, regardless of childhood vaccination status, because vaccine-induced immunity wanes with time, and even natural pertussis infection does not confer long-lasting immunity. Adolescents and adults with pertussis may have classic symptoms of whooping cough or may have only a lingering, mild cough.

Infants in the first year of life are at greatest risk for severe, life-threatening illness. They may lack maternally transferred antibodies during pregnancy and they will not have their own antibodies until they have received the standard vaccine series. This leaves infants vulnerable to pertussis throughout most of the first year of life. Infants are thought to have some protection once they complete the 3 dose primary DTaP vaccine series.

Mode of Spread ► Mode of spread is by the airborne route from aerosolized droplets generated by the intense cough of infected individuals. Much less often, infection may be acquired indirectly by handling objects freshly contaminated with nose and throat secretions. It is not thought that the *B. pertussis* bacteria can survive for very long on these objects though.

Incubation Period ► The incubation period is usually 7 to 10 days but may range from 5 to 21 days.

DIAGNOSIS

Culture of *B. pertussis* from secretions obtained from the posterior nose and throat by a through-the-nose swab remains the "gold standard" for laboratory diagnosis of pertussis in infants and children. *B. pertussis* is rarely cultured from adults.

Unfortunately, culture requires a minimum of 3 to 5 days for adequate growth for identification, and positive cultures are obtained in only 35 to 80 percent of patients with obvious clinical pertussis. Organisms are most likely to be recovered from patients in the catarrhal stage of illness when almost pure cultures may be obtained, particularly in very young infants. The diagnosis, however, is seldom suspected until the onset of the paroxysmal stage. After the first paroxysmal week, the likelihood of identifying the organism by culture decreases, and it is seldom possible to recover the organism from patients beyond 3 weeks after onset of the paroxysmal stage of illness. Positive cultures are also less likely in patients who have received antibiotic therapy with erythromycin, clarithromycin, azithromycin, or trimethoprim-sulfamethoxazole, or in vaccinated persons.

PCR testing is often used to detect *B. pertussis*. Pertussis PCR tests, which are sometimes available from your local or state health department, can be used to diagnose pertussis when the case also meets the clinical case definition (2 weeks of cough with paroxysms, inspiratory whoop, or post-cough vomiting). PCR has a higher sensitivity and shorter turnaround time than culture. When symptoms of classic pertussis are present (2 weeks of paroxysmal cough), PCR is 2 to 3 times more likely than culture to detect a positive *B. pertussis* sample. However, the accuracy of PCR-based *B. pertussis* tests vary widely among laboratories. The characteristic increased number of lymphocyte cells in the blood count seen with pertussis may be a helpful diagnostic aid, but it is nonspecific. Lymphocyte counts ranging from 20,000 to over 100,000 mm^3 are seen in the late catarrhal stage and throughout most of the paroxysmal stage. Lymphocytosis may not be present in children less than 6 months of age and in adults or partially immunized individuals.

TREATMENT

General Medical Management ► In addition to early diagnosis, experienced and efficient nursing care is probably the most important factor in survival of young infants with severe pertussis. Seventy percent of children who die of pertussis are less than 1 year of age and are most commonly 1 to 3 months of age. For this reason it is often wise to hospitalize younger infants until it can be determined that they don't have life-threatening paroxysms, apnea, cyanosis, or severe feeding problems. Children with these more severe symptoms may require frequent suctioning of secretions and oxygen administration during severe paroxysms. Parenteral fluid and electrolyte supplementation and, in protracted cases, intravenous feeding may be required.

Antimicrobial Agents ► Pertussis organisms are eradicated from patients with the disease if they are treated with antimicrobial agents active against B. *pertussis* organisms, provided that the drug diffuses in significant concentrations into respiratory tract secretions. No antimicrobial drug has been shown to alter the subsequent clinical course of the illness when given in the paroxysmal stage of the disease. However, drugs that meet these criteria do attenuate the illness when given in the catarrhal or pre-paroxysmal stage of the disease and abort or prevent the disease in individuals during incubation (asymptomatic susceptibles who are culture- or PCR-positive for B. *pertussis*). Their administration to patients at any stage of pertussis regularly produces bacteriologic cure and may render them non-infectious. These reasons constitute the rationale for the use of antimicrobials in pertussis. Macrolide antibiotics, including erythromycin, clarithromycin, and azithromycin, are the drugs of choice. Erythromycin is recommended for 14 days of therapy. Treatment for less than 14 days results in a 10 percent incidence of bacteriologic relapse, and these children may again become contagious. Trimethoprim-sulfamethoxazole is a possible alternative for patients who do not tolerate macrolides, but it is contraindicated for infants younger than 2 months of age. Clarithromycin and azithromycin for 7 days are the other macrolides that have been shown to be effective for treatment and chemoprophylaxis of pertussis, offering the advantage of shorter duration of treatment, less frequent dosing, and better tolerance.

Because of the risk of pyloric stenosis with erythromycin, azithromycin for 5 days is the drug of choice for treatment or post-exposure prophylaxis for pertussis in infants.

Children who develop fever or an elevated erythrocyte sedimentation rate usually have secondary suppurative infections, most often acute otitis media, sinusitis, or pneumonia. The bacterial pathogens implicated are those that usually cause these infections in infants and children, and thus require more targeted antimicrobial therapy.

Corticosteroids ▸ The usefulness of corticosteroids has not been demonstrated by any good studies and are not typically used to treat pertussis.

Albuterol ▸ Although a few small studies found that aerosolized albuterol treatments might be helpful in treating children with pertussis, another found no benefit, and it may not be worth the risk of agitating a child and triggering a coughing fit.

INFECTIOUS PERIOD

Individuals with pertussis should be considered infectious from just before the onset of the catarrhal stage of the disease until 3 weeks after the development of the paroxysmal cough or 5 days after starting effective antibiotic treatment.

INFECTION CONTROL

Parental Advice ▸ Parents should be told that pertussis or "whooping cough" has been diagnosed in children in the center and that measures have been taken to control the infection. These include isolation of infected individuals, pertussis vaccine administration to children who have not completed their immunization series, booster immunization for adult personnel, and antibiotic prophylaxis for all close contacts in the center. Parents should be instructed to watch for pertussis symptoms, to seek medical attention if their child develops any respiratory tract symptoms in the next 21 days, and to mention the possible pertussis exposure to their pediatrician.

Vaccine ▸ Effective control of pertussis depends on achieving universal immunization of infants and children and initiation of booster immunization for adolescents and adults. Infants and children should be immunized with a series of vaccinations containing diphtheria toxoid, tetanus toxoid, and acellular pertussis vaccine. Adolescents and adults who have received their recommended childhood vaccination series should receive booster immunization using a single dose of an age-appropriate tetanus toxoid, reduced diphtheria toxoid, and acellular pertussis vaccine (Tdap). Adults should receive a single Tdap booster immunization, even if they received the last dose of a tetanus toxoid–containing vaccine within the past 5 to 10 years. It is important that adults, including those aged 65 or older, who have or who anticipate having close contact with an infant 12 months of age or younger (e.g., parents, childcare providers, healthcare providers) receive a single dose of Tdap vaccine at least 1 month prior to close contact with the infant. Women should receive a dose of Tdap vaccine in the immediate postpartum period if they have not already been immunized. Any woman who might become pregnant is encouraged to receive a single dose of vaccine. Healthcare personnel who work in hospitals or ambulatory care settings and have direct patient contact should receive a single dose of vaccine. Close contacts of a newly infected patient should review their vaccination status. Those who are unimmunized or underimmunized, including children who are less than 10 years of age who have received fewer than four doses of their primary diphtheria, tetanus, and pertussis vaccines, and older children or adults who haven't had a Tdap booster, should be immunized in accordance with current recommended age-appropriate schedules.

Chemoprophylaxis ▶ All close contacts, including household and childcare contacts, who have been exposed to someone with pertussis should be considered infected and should receive chemoprophylaxis with an appropriate antibiotic, as outlined under Therapy, even if they are up-to-date on their vaccines. Chemoprophylaxis that is begun before or during the catarrhal phase may prevent or lessen illness.

Exclusion from Daycare or Preschool Attendance ▶ Children with symptomatic pertussis should be considered contagious from the earliest signs and symptoms of the catarrhal stage of illness to 3 weeks after onset of the paroxysmal stage. Nearly all children with pertussis who are treated with a macrolide antibiotic are culture-negative for *B. pertussis* organisms after 5 days, so that if compliance can be assured, these children may be considered non-contagious and return to the childcare setting after 5 days of antibiotics. However, treatment should be continued for at least 14 days if erythromycin is used and for 7 days if clarithromycin or azithromycin are used.

Recommendations for Other Children ▶ In addition to close contacts who are receiving prophylactic antibiotics, all children in a daycare center or preschool where pertussis has been confirmed in one or more children should be observed for pertussis symptoms for 21 days. Vaccine records should also be reviewed, and children without a complete vaccination series should be immunized.

Recommendations for Personnel ▶ When the diagnosis of pertussis has been confirmed in a daycare center, all exposed daycare center personnel should receive antibiotic prophylaxis with erythromycin, azithromycin, clarithromycin, or trimethoprim-sulfamethoxazole, and, if not fully vaccinated, be immunized with Tdap vaccine.

50

PNEUMOCOCCUS

(Otitis Media, Sinusitis, Bacteremia, Pneumonia, Meningitis)

Sheldon L. Kaplan

SIGNS AND SYMPTOMS

The most common diseases caused by *Streptococcus pneumoniae*, (also known as pneumococcus) are local respiratory infections such as ear infection and sinusitis, as well as invasive infections, including bloodstream infection, pneumonia, and meningitis. The incidence of invasive pneumococcal infections decreased dramatically after 2000 when immunization of all infants with the pneumococcal vaccine was recommended. The incidence of pneumococcal otitis media has decreased slightly as has the rate of tympanostomy tube placement. The pneumococcal serotypes included in the vaccine have almost been eliminated as a cause of invasive infections as well as otitis media. Serotypes not included in the vaccine now account for the vast majority of pneumococcal infections in children. In 2010, a 13-valent pneumococcal conjugate vaccine was approved and recommended for routine administration in infants and young children, thus increasing the serotypes that vaccinated children are protected against.

The pneumococcus is isolated from 30 to 40 percent of cases of otitis media and sinusitis in which a bacterial pathogen is identified. Pneumococcal otitis media frequently accompanies a viral respiratory infection. There are no clinical features that distinguish acute pneumococcal otitis media or sinusitis from infections with other germs. The pneumococcus can also cause conjunctivitis in young infants. Pneumonia is characterized by fever, tachypnea, localized findings on chest examination, and a pneumonia that involves one or more lobes seen on chest roentgenogram (X-ray). Symptoms usually improve dramatically after 1 or 2 days of appropriate antibacterial therapy.

The rate of bloodstream infection in otherwise healthy children between 3 and 36 months of age with temperatures above 39° C (102.2° F) for which no source can be identified has fallen to less than 1 percent in the *Haemophilus influenzae* type B and pneumococcal vaccine era. Nonetheless the pneumococcus continues to be the organism most often isolated from the blood of infants with bloodstream infection (bacteremia). Occult bacteremia is most often associated with upper respiratory infections, pharyngitis, or fever alone. Pneumococcal meningitis cannot be distinguished clinically from other types of bacterial meningitis.

CAUSE

The pneumococcus are lancet-shaped bacteria that are gram-positive cocci that occur in pairs. There are currently over 90 recognized serotypes.

SPREAD AND CONTROL

Source of the Organism ▶ *S. pneumoniae* are ubiquitous. Asymptomatic carriage of this organism is extremely common and carriage rates as high as 60 percent have been documented in young children. For adults living with children, the carriage rate approaches 20 to 30 percent, while the rate for adults without children in the household is only 6 percent. Pneumococci are often resistant to the most commonly used antibiotics in children. People recently treated with antibacterial agents and children attending daycare are more likely to be colonized with antibiotic-resistant pneumococci.

High-Risk Populations ► About 70 percent of pneumococcal infections in children occur in infants younger than 2 years old. Since the introduction of the vaccine, over 30 percent of children with systemic pneumococcal infections have underlying conditions. Children are considered at high or moderate risk for invasive pneumococcal infection if they have sickle cell disease, congenital or acquired lack of a spleen, splenic dysfunction, human immunodeficiency virus infection, congenital immune deficiency, chronic cardiac disease, chronic pulmonary disease, cerebrospinal fluid leak, chronic renal insufficiency or nephrotic syndrome, immunosuppressive chemotherapy, diabetes mellitus, or a cochlear implant.

Mode of Spread ► The pneumococcus spreads from person to person via respiratory droplets. Spread can occur in association with viral upper respiratory tract infections which are thought to be associated with increased adherence of the pneumococcus on respiratory epithelial cells.

Incubation Period ► There is no distinct incubation period for pneumococcal diseases. However, infection most often occurs within 1 month after an individual acquires a new serotype.

DIAGNOSIS

The diagnosis of infection caused by *S. pneumoniae* is usually made by isolation of the organism from body sites that are normally sterile (e.g., blood, spinal fluid). A diagnosis of pneumococcal pneumonia can be made by typical clinical and roentgenographic (X-ray) findings and the presence of gram-positive, lancet-shaped diplococcal bacteria in an adequate gram-stained sputum specimen, although sputum is difficult to obtain in children. Blood cultures may be positive in 5 to 10 percent of children hospitalized with pneumococcal pneumonia.

TREATMENT

Penicillin G remains the antibacterial agent of choice for most invasive infections caused by penicillin-susceptible *S. pneumoniae*. Otitis media, sinusitis, and pneumonia are often treated empirically with amoxicillin. Conjunctivitis can be treated with ophthalmic preparations of polymyxin B-bacitracin, sulfacetamide, or erythromycin. For children with life-threatening infection, namely meningitis, bacteremia, and pneumonia, the empiric use of ceftriaxone or cefotaxime plus vancomycin is recommended to cover antibiotic-resistant pneumococci as well other pathogens until isolates have been identified and antibiotic susceptibility information is available. The route of administration and whether the child is hospitalized will depend on the clinical setting. Pneumococci with reduced susceptibility to penicillin, cephalosporins, macrolides, clindamycin, and trimethoprim-sulfamethoxazole are being isolated with increasing frequency from children in daycare settings. Although the frequency of antibiotic resistance decreased following the introduction of the vaccine, resistance rates increased gradually several years later as serotype 19A became the most common serotype causing both local and invasive infections in children.

INFECTIOUS PERIOD

There is no evidence that children with *S. pneumoniae* infections are more likely to transmit the organism than are healthy children who are only carrying the bacteria.

INFECTION CONTROL

Parental Advice ▶ Nearly all children have *S. pneumoniae* in their upper respiratory tract at one time or another, and such "colonization" is seldom associated with disease. The fact that one child in the daycare center has an illness caused by *S. pneumoniae* probably does not increase the risk of another child having an illness with these bacteria. Children recently treated with antibacterial agents are more likely to have infections with pneumococci that have become more resistant to antibiotics than children who did not receive antibacterial therapy. Antibacterial agents should be used only when there are clear indications of bacterial infection. Antibacterial agents should not be used for colds, viral upper respiratory infections, bronchitis, or bronchiolitis.

Vaccine ▶ The 13-valent pneumococcal conjugate vaccine is recommended by the Advisory Committee on Immunization Practices and the American Academy of Pediatrics for universal administration to all infants.

The 23-valent pneumococcal polysaccharide vaccine (PPSV23) is recommended in addition to conjugate vaccine for children over 2 years of age who are at high risk for pneumococcal infection (e.g., children with sickle cell disease and children who have anatomic or functional asplenia, are immunocompromised, have human immunodeficiency virus infection, chronic cardiac disease, particularly cyanotic congenital heart disease, chronic pulmonary disease, chronic renal failure or nephrotic syndrome, asthma unless on high-dose corticosteroid therapy, cerebrospinal fluid leaks, cochlear implants, and diabetes mellitus). A second dose of PPSV23 is recommended 5 years after the first PPSV23 dose.

Exclusion from Daycare or Preschool Attendance ▶ Children should only be kept out of daycare or preschool if they are too ill to participate in usual activities.

Recommendations for Other Children ▶ Universal vaccination is recommended.

Recommendations for Personnel ▶ There are no recommendations for personnel in the daycare center once one child is known to be infected.

51

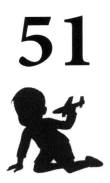

RESPIRATORY SYNCYTIAL VIRUS

(RSV)

Leigh B. Grossman

SIGNS AND SYMPTOMS

Respiratory syncytial virus (RSV) is the major cause of lower respiratory tract infection in infants and young children, and the most frequent cause of hospitalization in the first year of life. Bronchiolitis and pneumonia are the major manifestations during the first 2 years of life, and may vary in severity from mild to life-threatening or even fatal. Although essentially all first RSV infections cause symptoms, the vast majority of infants and young children have an uncomplicated course. Most at risk for severe and complicated disease are the very young infant and children with underlying diseases, especially those affecting the heart, lungs, and immune systems. Periods of not breathing, called apnea, may be a manifestation of RSV infection among infants within the first several months of life, particularly among premature infants. RSV is a major cause of tracheobronchitis among preschool-age children and occasionally may be manifest as croup. Close to half of primary infections are lower respiratory tract disease, and the other half are colds and ear infections.

RSV causes frequent and repetitive infections throughout life. Among children approximately 3 years of age or older, RSV infections are most often expressed as colds, ear infections, and croup. RSV is commonly associated with recurrent wheezing and occasionally may present as an influenza-like illness with fever. Adults may manifest recurrent RSV infection as bronchitis, wheezing, febrile upper respiratory tract infection, a cold, or with few symptoms. These mild infections are more apt to occur among those with recent or frequent exposure to children with RSV infections, such as personnel in childcare centers. Such mild infections may, nevertheless, be a source of spread of RSV.

CAUSE

RSV is an RNA virus. RSV strains are divided into two major groups, A and B. Given that there are 2 strains and immunity is not well understood, a child or adult can have repetitive RSV infections which can occur within a short time, even within the same season.

SPREAD AND CONTROL

Source of the Organism ▶ RSV is highly contagious and is spread from person to person. In the normal person, finding the virus in the secretions indicates an acute infection. Repetitive infections occasionally may be asymptomatic, but silent infection or carriage of the virus does not occur.

High-Risk Populations ▶ Young infants are most at risk for acquiring RSV infection and for developing severe disease. RSV occurs in annual outbreaks, primarily from November to April. Many children acquire RSV infection during their first winter season, and essentially all children experience RSV infection by 3 years of age. In daycare settings during the first year of life, the infection rate is especially high, sometimes almost all will become infected, and about half will have bronchiolitis or pneumonia. Even in the second and third year of life in childcare settings, two-thirds to three-fourths of the children will become infected with RSV. The reported rate of RSV infection is generally lower for children cared for at home than for those who are cared for in childcare settings, but, nevertheless, the infection rate is still high. Approximately two-thirds of the infants cared for at home in the first year of life have been shown to acquire RSV infection, and an even higher percentage have been shown to acquire RSV in the second year. During the third and fourth year of life, as many as one-third to one-half of children will become infected.

Children at risk for the most severe and complicated disease from RSV are those with premature birth, chronic lung disease, and cyanotic and functionally important congenital heart disease, compromised immunity, and congenital anomalies or neurologic diseases that affect pulmonary function or may predispose to gastroesophageal reflux and aspiration. Older children with asthma disease may have exacerbations of wheezing and more prolonged illness.

Mode of Spread ► RSV is spread by direct contact with infectious secretions. This appears to be primarily by large-particle aerosols from infected individuals within close proximity and from contact with infectious secretions on environmental surfaces. The infectious secretions on surfaces, toys, clothes, and other objects are transmitted by touching, with subsequent self-inoculation of the virus by touching the eyes or nose. RSV may remain infectious on the skin for about a half an hour and on surfaces for as long as a day or more, depending on the temperature, humidity, and type of surface.

Incubation Period ► The incubation period ranges from 3 to 7 days but most frequently appears to be 3 to 5 days.

DIAGNOSIS

The season, age, and clinical presentation, especially bronchiolitis, allow a presumptive diagnosis in many infants. Specific diagnostic tests performed on respiratory secretions include rapid antigen and molecular assays, and viral isolation, which usually requires 3 to 7 days. Detection by polymerase chain reaction (PCR) in respiratory secretions is highly sensitive and specific and is now widely available.

TREATMENT

Most children attending daycare who acquire RSV infection require no more than the usual supportive care for an upper respiratory tract infection. Some may benefit from fever-reducing medication, although fever associated with RSV infection is usually not high and does not correlate with the severity of the illness.

An appreciable proportion of these children also may manifest wheezing, which may be intermittent and variable in severity, from mild enough to be detectable only on auscultation, to severe with respiratory distress. Bronchodilators, mostly nebulized, are frequently used, but for most children with acute RSV infection, especially young infants with a first episode of wheezing, bronchodilators are not recommended as they provide little or no benefit and may be associated with adverse effects.

For more severely ill children requiring hospitalization, supportive care remains the mainstay of therapy. Ribavirin may be considered for use in children with severe illness or with high-risk underlying conditions.

INFECTIOUS PERIOD

RSV is shed in the respiratory secretions of young infants for 1 to 2 weeks but occasionally may be longer. In older children and adults, shedding of the virus is less, usually 3 to 7 days.

INFECTION CONTROL

Parental Advice ▶ Parents should be informed about the prevalence and contagiousness of RSV among young children in any setting during a community outbreak of RSV infection. They should understand that all children acquire RSV infection in the first few years of life, and if the child is over 1 year of age or has been in the daycare center through a previous RSV season, the child is highly likely to have already experienced RSV infection. Thus, if their child acquires a respiratory infection, they should treat it as any other respiratory illness and seek the advice of their physician.

Vaccine ▶ None.

Prophylaxis ▶ An antibody directed against the RSV (palivizumab) has been licensed for prevention in a select group of premature high-risk infants and those with chronic cardiopulmonary diseases. Palivizumab may be administered intramuscularly once per month, for up to five months, during the RSV season. In controlled studies, palivizumab prophylaxis has resulted in a significant reduction in the risk of hospitalizations. Palivizumab does not prevent upper respiratory tract infections, and thus, children receiving prophylaxis may still be infectious from RSV infection.

Exclusion from Daycare or Preschool Attendance ▶ Because of the ubiquitous and prevalent nature of RSV during a winter community outbreak, and because the clinical presentation may be variable and not distinguishable from respiratory illnesses caused by many other pathogens, preventing an infected child from attending a daycare or preschool setting is impractical in most instances. Furthermore, children may be highly infectious just prior to the onset of symptoms. For those children known to have RSV infection, particularly with lower respiratory tract infection, the best guideline for return to the childcare setting is when the child is clinically well enough to be able to attend and participate in the usual activities.

Recommendations for Other Children ▶ Studies have shown that once one child in a daycare or preschool setting is infected, spread of RSV infection is often rapid and inevitable. Also, children frequently acquire RSV infection outside of the daycare setting during a community outbreak. Routine hand cleansing procedures by washing and use of hand sanitizers is probably the most effective means of protection against the spread of RSV infection, and should be consistently practiced by personnel in the daycare center. Although enforcing good hand cleansing among children is difficult, emphasis on routine hand cleaning in daycare centers has been shown to result in fewer respiratory and gastrointestinal illnesses.

Communal toys and equipment should be routinely cleaned, and, when possible, toys should be assigned to individual child use.

Recommendations for Personnel ► Personnel in a daycare center or preschool frequently become infected with RSV, which most often is manifest as an upper respiratory tract infection. Nevertheless, they may serve as disseminators of RSV infection to others in the center. As RSV is spread primarily by direct contact with infectious secretions, which may remain contagious on skin and environmental surfaces for some time, good and constant hand cleansing is integral to controlling RSV transmission. Personnel with upper respiratory infections, if possible, should not work while acutely symptomatic. In addition, personnel should be educated as to the modes of spread of RSV, and the recommendations for prevention of spread of respiratory infections should be periodically reviewed.

52

RHINOVIRUSES

(Common Cold)

Ronald B. Turner

SIGNS AND SYMPTOMS

The rhinoviruses are an important cause of the common cold. The symptoms of rhinovirus colds are limited to the upper respiratory tract in most people; fever or muscle aches and pains are uncommon. Gastrointestinal symptoms are not associated with rhinovirus infections. The first symptom noted by many individuals is a mild sore throat. This is soon followed by development of nasal stuffiness and a runny nose. About one-third of rhinovirus illnesses are associated with cough. Symptoms reach a peak after 1 to 2 days of illness and usually resolve within 7 to 10 days.

Although rhinovirus infection is usually minor and self-limited, a small proportion of infected individuals will have complications. Rhinovirus colds may be complicated by an ear infection due to either the rhinovirus itself or a secondary bacterial infection. Sinusitis may also complicate the viral infection. Lower respiratory symptoms, especially exacerbations of asthma, are reported in about 1 percent of these infections.

CAUSE

The rhinoviruses are RNA viruses. There are more than 100 different serotypes of rhinovirus.

SPREAD AND CONTROL

Source of the Organism ► Infection with the rhinoviruses is acquired exclusively from other infected individuals. There is no animal host for this virus. The virus can survive on inanimate objects for several hours, and contaminated objects can presumably serve as a source of infection.

High-Risk Populations ► There is no population that is known to be at increased risk of infection with the rhinoviruses. Patients with asthma may be at risk of more severe asthma symptoms if infection with rhinovirus occurs.

Mode of Spread ► Spread of rhinovirus infection has been demonstrated to occur by direct contact, via contaminated objects, and in aerosols. The relative importance of these different routes of spread in the natural setting is not known.

Incubation Period ► The incubation period for rhinovirus infection is 1 to 2 days.

DIAGNOSIS

Rhinovirus illnesses are generally mild, and making a specific etiologic diagnosis is not generally attempted. Laboratory diagnosis is accomplished by isolation of the organism in cell culture and by polymerase chain reaction (PCR) tests.

TREATMENT

There are no anti-infective therapies of proven benefit for treatment of rhinovirus infections. Cold symptoms can be treated with over-the-counter medications in children over 4 years of age. Topical decongestant therapies are the most efficacious. Antihistamines have a modest effect on the runny nose and cough associated with colds; however, drowsiness is a frequent side effect.

INFECTIOUS PERIOD

Infected individuals may shed virus in nasal secretions for as long as 3 weeks. Transmission is most likely when nasal symptoms are present.

INFECTION CONTROL

Parental Advice ▸ No special measures are indicated.

Vaccine ▸ None available.

Exclusion from Daycare or Preschool Attendance ▸ Exclusion of rhinovirus-infected children from childcare settings is not indicated.

Recommendations for Other Children ▸ Transmission of infection may be reduced by frequent handwashing.

Recommendations for Personnel ▸ Transmission of infection may be reduced by frequent handwashing.

53

ROSEOLA

(Exanthema Subitum)

J. Christopher Day
Mary Anne Jackson

SIGNS AND SYMPTOMS

Roseola (also called exanthema subitum) is the most common fever and rash illness in children ages 6 months to 2 years and is typically caused by human herpes virus 6 (HHV-6) or, in some cases, HHV-7 infection. In typical cases, high, sustained fever is present and lasts for 3 to 5 days. Irritability, malaise, and runny nose may be present during this time, but usually, despite the high fever, most children are alert and playful. A red throat with small lesions on the palate or tonsils may be seen in 65 percent of patients, and lymph node swelling in the posterior neck and behind the ears may be the only other pertinent findings. Children with roseola may have eyelid swelling that gives them a "sleepy" or "droopy" appearance. Many clinicians believe this is a classic pre-rash finding, although it occurs in only 30 percent of infants with roseola.

The exanthem or rash phase of roseola generally occurs co-incident with the disappearance of fever. Exanthema sub-itum means "sudden rash" in Latin. Pale rose-pink macules measuring 2 to 5 millimeters are surrounded by a white halo and scattered over the neck and trunk, sparing the face and extremities. The rash lasts 24 to 48 hours, and a total clinical course of 5 to 7 days is typical.

High fever without localizing signs occurs frequently. In one survey, rash was noted in less than 20 percent of febrile children visiting the Emergency Department with primary HHV-6 infection. Another population-based study suggests that the acquisition of HHV-6 in infancy often results in fever, fussiness, diarrhea, rash, or classic roseola presentation. Medical evaluation in such children is common: nearly 4 in 10 will visit a physician. Febrile seizures and other neurologic manifestations of roseola may require further evaluation and other diagnostic studies. In the United Kingdom, 26 (17 percent) of 205 children 2 months old to 35 months old who were prospectively followed and hospitalized for suspected encephalitis or severe illness with fever and seizures had HHV-6 or -7 infection. Hospitalization averaged 7 days with almost half requiring intensive care. Fatal liver failure has been described in an infant with primary HHV-6 infection.

Primary infection in adults can present with a mononucleosis-type illness. Various neurologic manifestations, including encephalitis, are well described in both immunocompromised hosts as well as in immunocompetent adults and are typically associated with reactivated disease.

Fever, hepatitis, pneumonia, and bone marrow suppression have also been reported in immunocompromised hosts in whom reactivation has occurred. An association with graft rejection has been noted in liver and kidney transplant patients.

CAUSE

HHV-6 and -7 are DNA viruses first described in 1986 and 1990, respectively. These pathogens are ubiquitous and acquired early in life.

HHV-6 infection is most common; primary infection occurs in 40 percent of infants in the first year of life, in 77 percent by age 2, and approach 100 percent by age 3 years. Two variants of HHV-6 are recognized (A and B), with primary infection with HHV-6B causing most cases of roseola. HHV-6 appears to establish latent infection by integrating into the cellular DNA, a unique mechanism among human herpes viruses. Primary HHV-7 infection appears to occur slightly later in life. Twenty percent of healthy children are seropositive by 1 year, 40 percent by 2 years, 50 percent by 3 years, and greater than 90 percent of adults demonstrate evidence of past infections.

At times, roseola-like illness has been associated with other viruses including enteroviruses (most commonly ECHO-16 virus), adenoviruses, and parvovirus.

SPREAD AND CONTROL

Source of the Organism ▸ The human is the only known host for roseola. There is no distinct seasonality.

High-Risk Populations ▸ Reactivated disease has been reported in immunocompromised hosts.

Mode of Spread ▸ Contact with the infected saliva of healthy persons is the probable mode of spread. Older siblings and parents are the usual source of this virus for the first infection in their young children.

Incubation Period ▸ Nine to 10 days.

DIAGNOSIS

Although such testing is not universally available, HHV-6 and -7 can be isolated from blood and detected by polymerase chain reaction (PCR) which is most often utilized in the immunocompromised population. In an otherwise healthy child, laboratory confirmation of acute infection is not generally needed. Antibody testing has shown to be a reliable discriminator between HHV-6 and -7.

Diagnosis of roseola is generally made on clinical grounds. The diagnosis is established by documenting a pattern of fever followed by the typical rash at the time the fever disappears.

TREATMENT

Treatment is supportive. While ganciclovir, foscarnet, or sometimes cidofovir may be considered in severe disease in the compromised patient, there are no prospective studies to confirm efficacy.

INFECTIOUS PERIOD

The period of communicability is unknown. It appears likely that individuals with asymptomatic reactivations of disease are the source of most infections.

INFECTION CONTROL

Parental Advice ▶ Cases usually occur sporadically throughout the year. Occasionally outbreaks have been reported, but parents can be reassured as to the benign nature of this infection. There is no known risk to pregnant women, and roseola in children less than 3 months or children over 4 years of age is uncommon.

Vaccine ▶ None available.

Exclusion from Daycare or Preschool Attendance ▶ Generally speaking, children with febrile rashes should not return to a daycare or preschool setting until their rash is gone and they are well. No exclusion is necessary for laboratory-proven HHV-6 or HHV-7 disease.

Recommendations for Other Children ▶ No contact prophylaxis is necessary.

Recommendations for Personnel ▶ No special recommendations are necessary for childcare personnel.

54

ROTAVIRUS

Theresa A. Schlager

SIGNS AND SYMPTOMS

Rotavirus infection is the most common cause of gastroenteritis occurring in the winter among infants and young children in the United States. The clinical features of rotavirus infection vary from asymptomatic fecal shedding of the virus to severe vomiting and diarrhea associated with dehydration and shock. Symptomatic illness usually is manifested by vomiting and low-grade fever followed by watery, nonbloody diarrhea. Vomiting and dehydration occur more frequently with rotavirus infection than with other causes of gastroenteritis. Diarrhea typically lasts between 3 and 8 days but may be prolonged in immunocompromised children. Respiratory symptoms are associated with rotavirus, but the virus has not been isolated from respiratory secretions. The overall course of rotavirus infection ordinarily is self-limited and with full recovery if appropriate therapy for dehydration is provided.

CAUSE

Rotaviruses are RNA viruses and there are at least seven distinct groups (A to G). Group A is the major cause of infantile diarrhea. Five strains account for over 90 percent of clinical illness in developed countries; however, strain distribution may be more diverse in developing countries. Thus, an effective vaccine must provide protection against several strains that a child may be exposed to. Rotavirus appears to cause disease by invading and altering small bowel mucosal cells, resulting in malabsorption and diarrhea.

SPREAD AND CONTROL

Source of the Organism ▶ Rotavirus is one of the most common causes of diarrhea in the childcare center for children younger than 4 years of age and represents a source of infection for parents and childcare providers. Among the many viruses causing diarrhea, rotavirus is one of the most common causes of severe illness. Although symptomatic disease in adults is unusual, asymptomatic shedding of the virus by adults can be a source of infection. Animals are known to have rotavirus diarrheal disease, but animal-to-human transmission has not been documented under natural conditions.

High-Risk Populations ▶ The peak age for symptomatic rotavirus infection is 6 to 24 months, and virtually all children are infected by 3 years of age. The disease is highly contagious, and contact with infected patients in the 6- to 24-month-old age group constitutes the greatest risk factor for disease acquisition. The immunocompromised child is at risk for developing chronic diarrhea. Reinfections are usually milder than the primary infection.

Mode of Spread ▶ Fecal–oral spread is the most common mode of spread, but contaminated environmental surfaces and objects may also transmit rotavirus.

Incubation Period ▶ One to 3 days.

DIAGNOSIS

Although a specific diagnosis is usually not necessary, a very good rapid diagnostic antibody test for group A rotovirus is available.

Fresh stool specimens from the first 4 days of illness have the highest yield for rotavirus detection and correlate with the highest degree of viral shedding. The presence of detectable rotavirus in feces usually correlates with acute diarrheal symptoms. In some patients, rotavirus may be shed for as long as 3 weeks, thereby permitting a diagnosis well after the initial onset of diarrhea.

TREATMENT

No specific antiviral therapy is available. Adequate fluid replacement is the mainstay of treatment. Most patients can be managed appropriately with oral rehydration, but infants with marked dehydration may require hospitalization for intravenous fluid and electrolyte repletion. In one study, lactobacillus GG, a probiotic, significantly reduced the duration of acute rotaviral gastroenteritis in children with normal immune function. The routine use of oral immunoglobulin for rotavirus gastroenteritis has not proved to be beneficial when compared to rehydration therapy alone. However, in immunodeficient children with chronic rotavirus infection, orally administered rotavirus-specific immunoglobulin preparations may ablate shedding or lesson disease symptoms.

INFECTIOUS PERIOD

The infectious period is usually less than 1 week, paralleling diarrhea that usually ceases in 4 to 5 days. However, severe rotavirus disease in young and immunocompromised patients may be followed by extended excretion of rotavirus.

INFECTION CONTROL

Parental Advice ▶ A daycare center or preschool should notify parents of children who have been in direct contact with a child who has diarrhea. Parents should contact their physician for advice if their child develops diarrhea.

Breastfeeding ▶ Breast milk antibodies coat infant mucosal surfaces and may play a role in protecting infants from infection by pathogens such as rotavirus that have a mucosal site of entry.

Vaccine ▸ The first vaccine was licensed in the United States in 1999 and withdrawn 9 months later due to reports of an association between the vaccine and intussusception (bowel obstruction). Subsequently, two orally administered rotavirus vaccines have demonstrated efficacy in preventing gastroenteritis and resulted in lower rates of infant hospitalization. Studies to date have demonstrated no difference in the rates of intussusception between vaccine and placebo groups. In 2006, the Advisory Committee on Immunization Practices (ACIP) to the Centers for Disease Control and Prevention (CDC) recommended that all infants receive the oral vaccine.

Exclusion from Daycare or Preschool Attendance ▸ The infected child should be kept out of the daycare or preschool setting as long as diarrhea or vomiting is present.

Recommendations for Other Children ▸ Routine testing for rotavirus in other children who have been exposed within a daycare center or preschool is not recommended. Washing of children's hands on arrival at the center, after a diaper change or use of the toilet, and before meals and snacks should be consistently practiced. Use of liquid soap in a dispenser along with disposable paper towels is recommended. Rotaviruses are inactivated by 70 percent ethanol, which is the preferred solution for cleaning contaminated surfaces.

Recommendations for Personnel ▸ Symptomatic staff members should not attend the center until fever, diarrhea, or vomiting ceases. Without failure, staff members should practice careful hand washing (10 seconds with soap and warm running water) upon arrival at the center, after changing a child's diaper, after using or providing assistance to a child using the toilet, and before food handling. Disinfecting diaper-changing surfaces along with proper diaper disposal is recommended.

55

RUBELLA

(German Measles)

Gregory F. Hayden

SIGNS AND SYMPTOMS

Rubella (German measles) is commonly inapparent and unrecognized. When clinical illness occurs, it is generally benign and is manifested by rash and lymphadenopathy with mild constitutional symptoms. The pink, raised rash appears first on the face and then spreads downward and then out to the arms and legs. The usual duration of rash is 2 to 5 days, leading to the lay term "3-day measles." The illness is often more severe among adolescents and adults whose illness may begin with a prodrome or early phase of fever, malaise, headache, and respiratory symptoms. Arthralgia and arthritis may occur, especially in adult women. Rare complications include thrombocytopenic purpura (decrease in platelet numbers and vascular inflammation) and encephalitis.

In contrast to the usually mild nature of rubella occurring after birth, rubella occurring in the unborn baby can be devastating. Virtually every organ system can be affected, but especially the eyes, heart, and central nervous system. The clinical expression of congenital rubella depends on the timing of infection, with the risk of major anomalies being greatest during the first trimester.

CAUSE

Rubella is an RNA virus. Only one serologic type is recognized.

SPREAD AND CONTROL

Reported rubella has declined substantially since the rubella vaccine was licensed in 1969. Fewer than 25 cases of rubella have been reported in the United States each year since 2001, and rubella is no longer considered endemic. It remains important, however, to maintain high immunization rates among children and to respond rapidly to any outbreak.

Source of the Organism ► The human is the only known natural host and source of infection.

High-Risk Populations ► Rubella is uncommon in the first several months of life when babies still have some maternal antibody protection, but after this age, unvaccinated children remain at high risk of developing rubella if exposed.

Mode of Spread ► Transmission is via respiratory droplets or direct contact with an infected patient.

Incubation Period ► The incubation period is usually 16 to 18 days but can range from 14 to 23 days.

DIAGNOSIS

The clinical diagnosis of postnatal rubella can be confirmed by viral culture or antibody tests. The rubella virus can be isolated from the nose, throat, and other sites, but viral culture is relatively expensive and not universally available. Polymerase chain reaction (PCR) testing is available. Several serologic techniques that document an antibody response to the virus are available. A suspected or confirmed diagnosis of rubella should be reported immediately to the local health department.

TREATMENT

No specific therapy is currently available.

INFECTIOUS PERIOD

The period of maximum communicability occurs from up to 5 days before rash onset until 5 to 7 days after rash onset. More rarely, virus has been detected in the nose and throat as long as 7 days before and 14 days after rash onset.

INFECTION CONTROL

Parental Advice ▶ Parents should be advised that a suspected (or confirmed) case of rubella has occurred in a child at the center. They should be advised that the risk to their child is minimal so long as he or she has already received rubella vaccine. Parents of unimmunized children should be advised to seek medical advice immediately concerning the prompt vaccination of children over 1 year of age and concerning the potential risk their child may pose to susceptible pregnant contacts. Parents should also be urged to verify their own immunity status as well as the immunization status of any older children, especially adolescents, who do not attend the center, and to seek vaccination as appropriate. A mother who is pregnant should discuss this possible exposure with her obstetrician.

Vaccine ▶ Live, attenuated rubella virus vaccine should be given routinely to children after the first birthday, and is usually administered at 12 to 15 months of age as a part of the combined measles-mumps-rubella (MMR) vaccine or the combined measles-mumps-rubella-varicella (MMRV) vaccine. The cornerstone of rubella prevention in daycare centers and preschools should be the vigilant insistence that all children 15 months of age or older have received rubella vaccine as a pre-requisite for attending the center. A single dose confers long-lasting rubella immunity to more than 90 percent of vaccinees, but a second dose at 4 to 6 years of age maximizes the rate of immunity and provides an added safeguard against primary vaccine failures.

Precautions and contraindications to live rubella vaccination include altered immunity, pregnancy, severe febrile illness, and recent administration of an immune globulin preparation or blood products. Children with minor illnesses, with or without fever, may be vaccinated. MMR vaccine is recommended for children infected with the human immunodeficiency virus (HIV) if they are not severely immunocompromised.

Exclusion from Daycare or Preschool Attendance ▶ Children with postnatal rubella should be excluded from daycare or preschool for 7 days after rash onset. As patients are often contagious before rash onset, however, and because inapparent infections can be communicable, attempts to control spread by means of isolation are commonly ineffective.

Children with congenital rubella should be considered contagious until they are one year old, unless nose, throat, and urine cultures after 3 months of age are repeatedly negative for rubella.

Recommendations for Other Children ▶ The first step is to verify that other children attending the center have already been immunized against rubella in accordance with established center policy. Children with documented previous immunization against rubella are highly unlikely to develop illness and may continue to attend the center. The management of unvaccinated children is more complex. Live rubella vaccine is not known to prevent illness when given after exposure, but theoretically it can prevent illness if administered within 3 days of exposure, and it will at least protect against subsequent exposures if the child is not already incubating wild rubella infection. Immunization of a child who is incubating natural rubella is not known to be harmful. For unvaccinated children who have reached their first birthday, vaccination can therefore be recommended. Parents must understand, however, that the vaccine may not block the progression of incubating rubella, so that they will not wrongly blame the vaccine for rubella illness that develops after vaccination.

For infants younger than 1 year of age, vaccination is a less attractive option because the likelihood of developing protective antibodies is believed to be lower. Although limited data suggest that it can potentially prevent or modify infection in exposed susceptibles, immunoglobulin is not generally recommended in this instance because of its expense, its questionable efficacy, and the usually mild clinical course of rubella in young children.

Recommendations for Personnel ► Ideally, all staff members should provide a documented history of immunization or serologic evidence of immunity at the time of employment. Strict adherence to such a policy will reduce or eliminate the needless disruption that can arise among personnel when rubella is diagnosed in a child attending the center. If appropriate preparations have not been made before such a case occurs, the first step is to determine whether any staff members are susceptible to rubella. This determination is particularly crucial for any personnel who may possibly be pregnant. Documented history of previous rubella immunization on or after the first birthday strongly suggests immunity to rubella. The detection of antibody by a properly performed test before or at the time of exposure provides strong evidence that the individual is immune and not at risk for developing rubella. If antibody is not detectable immediately after an exposure of rubella, additional blood testing will be necessary to determine whether infection has occurred. A pregnant woman exposed to rubella should consult her obstetrician immediately to discuss and evaluate the possible implications of this exposure. In most instances, the woman will already be immune to rubella and can be reassured that the exposure poses little or no risk to her developing fetus.

56

RUBEOLA

(Measles)

Leigh B. Grossman

SIGNS AND SYMPTOMS

The onset of rubeola is usually 8 to 12 days after exposure and characteristically consists of fever and the "three C's"– coryza (runny nose), conjunctivitis (pinkeye), and cough. After 3 to 4 days, the rash first appears. The typical red raised rash starts on the head, around the hairline, and progresses to the feet over 3 days, changing from discrete lesions to a confluent rash. About 2 days prior to the onset of the rash the typical white Koplik spots may appear on the cheek or buccal mucosa inside the mouth. Once the rash appears, the respiratory symptoms and fever disappear. The rash fades over the subsequent several days, leaving a brown stain followed by a generalized peeling that has the appearance of bran. Classic measles generally resolves over a 10-day period, but the cough may persist. Cough, ear infection, croup, and pneumonia may complicate the course of rubeola.

The severity of the disease and mortality rates are increased among preschool children and immunocompromised children, such as those with cancer or human immunodeficiency virus

(HIV) infection. Among immunocompromised children, the rash may be uncharacteristic or even absent, resulting in the diagnosis being unsuspected.

Clinical variants of classic measles include modified measles, atypical measles, and vaccine measles. Modified measles is a mild form of measles with a shortened course occurring in patients who possess some measles antibody, such as those who have received gamma globulin, occasionally in infants who still have some antibody from their mother, and about 5 percent may have waning immunity after vaccination. Atypical measles is a severe and clinically unusual form of measles which was observed in patients who previously had received inactivated measles vaccine, which ceased to be marketed after 1968. After exposure to the wild virus these patients developed a high fever, sometimes a nodular pneumonia, and an unusual rash that could be petechial, vesicular, nodular, or urticarial, as well as macular-papular. Cough and conjunctivitis were uncommon. With widespread use of live vaccine, this atypical disease is no longer seen. Vaccine measles is the usually mild illness that appears in some children 7 to 12 days following administration of the attenuated vaccine. Fever occurs in about 15 percent of children receiving the vaccine and a transient rash develops in about 5 percent.

Acute encephalitis may be associated with measles in approximately 0.1 percent of cases. Subacute sclerosing panencephalitis (SSPE) is a late neurologic complication of measles which occurred in approximately 1 in 100,000 cases, but has essentially disappeared in the United States and in other areas where measles vaccine administration is routine.

CAUSE

Measles virus is an RNA virus.

SPREAD AND CONTROL

Source of the Organism ▶ Measles is spread from person to person, and humans are the only source of the virus, although monkeys may be infected with measles.

High-Risk Populations ▶ Measles is highly contagious, and nonimmune individuals are at high risk of acquiring infection in areas where measles is common. Infants, pregnant women, adults, and those with underlying diseases, especially immunocompromising conditions, including HIV, tend to be at increased risk for severe and complicated disease.

Mode of Spread ▶ Measles is spread by contact with secretions of infected persons. Infectious secretions may be spread by large-particle droplets, requiring close contact, or less commonly by small-particle aerosols that may allow rapid and distant transmission of the virus. Self-inoculation after direct contact with infectious secretions on contaminated environmental surfaces or objects may also occur. An infected individual should be considered infectious by the airborne route through 4 days after the appearance of the rash. Inoculation appears to occur via the nose, throat, and mucosa of the eye.

Incubation Period ▶ The incubation period is usually 8 to 12 days.

DIAGNOSIS

Diagnosis is often made clinically in the classic case. Confirmation of the diagnosis of measles may be made by isolation of the virus from secretions, by tissue culture, or by tests that document an antibody response to measles virus infection. Diagnosis by polymerase chain reaction (PCR) on specimens of blood and secretions is also available and is highly sensitive and specific.

TREATMENT

Measles is usually a self-limited disease, and therapy is mainly supportive. The antiviral drug ribavirin has been shown in the laboratory to have activity against measles virus. In controlled studies in children in other countries, oral ribavirin therapy has appeared to shorten the course of the disease. In the United States, aerosolized and intravenous ribavirin has been used for severe measles pneumonia, but the experience is limited, and the drug is not approved for this use.

Vitamin A treatment of children with measles in developing countries has resulted in diminished measles severity and mortality, and thus is recommended by the World Health Organization to be administered to all children with measles in areas where vitamin A deficiency exists and where the mortality from measles is 1 percent or more. In the United States, vitamin A deficiency generally is not a problem, but low vitamin A levels have been documented in the blood of some children with severe measles. The American Academy of Pediatrics, therefore, recommends that vitamin A supplementation be considered for children 6 months to 2 years of age with measles severe enough to require hospitalization and for those children 6 months of age or older who have certain risk factors, such as those with immunodeficiency, nutritional problems, including impaired intestinal absorption, and for children from areas in other countries in which measles mortality is high.

Antibiotics should be used only for proven bacterial complications of measles, such as ear infection or pneumonia.

INFECTIOUS PERIOD

Measles is considered to be contagious from 1 to 2 days before the onset of symptoms, usually 3 to 5 days before the onset of the rash, to 3 to 4 days after its appearance. In immuno-compromised children, the duration of viral shedding and, thus, ability to spread the virus is prolonged. Measles is most infectious during the "cold" stage when it is most difficult to diagnose. Once the rash appears, the communicability of the disease rapidly declines.

INFECTION CONTROL

Parental Advice ► Parents of children attending a daycare center or preschool in which measles has occurred should be immediately notified, and the recommendations for their children, as stated above, should be given to them in written form, and they should be urged to consult their physician immediately. The importance and urgency of this should be stressed, and the contagiousness of measles emphasized. The parents also should understand that children who are susceptible and those who do not comply with the above recommendations will have to be excluded from daycare or preschool until the risk of the spread of measles is over, which may mean 4 weeks from the time of the onset of the last case.

Vaccine ▶ In the United States, 2 combination vaccines are available, measles-mumps-rubella vaccine (MMR) and measles-mumps-rubella-varicella vaccine (MMRV). Monovalent measles vaccine is no longer available in the United States. MMR or MMRV is recommended routinely for all children at 12 to 15 months of age. A second dose of measles vaccine, MMR or MMRV, should be administered routinely at the time of school entry. In special circumstances, such as during outbreaks or international travel, the vaccine may be administered earlier, as long as the first and second doses are separated by at least 4 weeks. During measles outbreaks, the initial measles immunization may be given to children as young as 6 months of age. Children receiving their initial vaccination before the first birthday should be revaccinated at 12 to 15 months of age, and a third dose should be administered at 4 to 6 years of age.

Exclusion from Daycare or Preschool Attendance ▶ A child with a known or suspected case of measles should be excluded from the daycare or preschool setting through 4 days after the onset of the rash.

Recommendations for Other Children ▶ If a case of measles is suspected in a childcare center, the local health department should be notified immediately. In a daycare center or preschool in which measles has occurred, a program of revaccination with MMR is recommended. Unvaccinated children who are 6 months of age or older also should receive the live measles vaccine. If the vaccine is given within 72 hours of exposure, it may give protection against infection. Immunoglobulin can be administered to unvaccinated children within 6 days of exposure. If the immunoglobulin is given at doses larger than 0.25 ml/kg, measles vaccine must be delayed for 5 months or longer.

Recommendations for Personnel ▶ As susceptible adults are at risk for severe measles infection, it is essential that personnel exposed in a daycare or preschool setting know their immunization status, preferably at the time of employment. Although recommendations specific for this setting do not exist, the recommendations for those in medical facilities and for young adults in the college setting are that at the time of employment or enrollment they must have proof of immunity or proof of having had two doses of vaccine. Similar recommendations would seem advisable for personnel in the child-care setting who were born after 1956. Once measles has been introduced into the daycare or preschool setting, all adults who do not have clear proof of having had measles disease or of having received two doses of the vaccine should be immunized, especially if born after 1956.

57

SALMONELLA

Linda A. Waggoner-Fountain

SIGNS AND SYMPTOMS

Diseases caused by salmonella can be classified into four categories: typhoid fever, enteric fever, focal infection, and diarrheal disease.

Typhoid fever is a multisystem illness that may or may not be associated with diarrhea. Enteric fever is the syndrome of diarrhea and high fever often associated with bloodstream infection. Following bacteremia, which may or may not be symptomatic, salmonella organisms can localize in virtually any organ of the body and cause focal infection. The most common are meningitis, skeletal infections, urinary tract infections, and gallbladder disease.

Gastrointestinal syndromes take several forms. The most common is a mild to moderately severe diarrheal illness with abdominal pain, tenesmus (the urgent need to defecate), and fever. The illness resolves spontaneously within a few days. When heavily contaminated food is ingested, a food poisoning syndrome ensues that is characterized principally by repeated vomiting over a few hours. On occasion, salmonella causes colitis with a dysentery (bloody diarrhea) syndrome identical to that seen with shigella. Finally, a failure-to-thrive syndrome occurs in some young infants who have smoldering salmonella enteritis without frank diarrhea.

CAUSE

Salmonella organisms are gram-negative enteric bacilli. Typhoid fever syndrome is caused by *Salmonella typhi, S. paratyphi A, S. paratyphi B*, and *S. choleraesuis. S. typhimurium* and *S. enteritidis* are the most common species causing gastroenteritis.

SPREAD AND CONTROL

Source of the Organism ▶ In typhoid fever, the human is the principal reservoir of infection, whereas in other salmonella infections domestic animals, especially chickens, are the reservoir. Pet turtles were a common source of infection until laws were enacted to control the problem. Iguanas, snakes, and other reptiles remain a potential reservoir of infection. Salmonellosis is more common in the summer months.

High-Risk Populations ▶ Children have the highest incidence of salmonellosis: Young children, the elderly and the immunocompromised are most likely to develop severe infection when infected.

Mode of Spread ▶ Person-to-person spread can occur, but this mode is very unusual except in the case of immunocompromised individuals. The usual source of infection is contaminated food. Eggs and products containing raw eggs are especially high-risk foods. Because healthy individuals are resistant to small numbers of salmonella germs, improper cooking and storage of contaminated foods under conditions that promote growth of the organism are important epidemiologic factors. There have been numerous epidemics of salmonella infection from common source-contaminated foods including fresh produce (sprouts, hot peppers, tomatoes, lettuce, melons) and a variety of other foods including spices such as black and white pepper, peanut butter, chocolate and dried milk. Person-to-person spread has not been a major problem in childcare centers.

Incubation Period ► The incubation period is from 6 to 72 hours for gastroenteritis and from 7 to 14 days for typhoid fever.

DIAGNOSIS

The diagnosis of gastroenteritis is by culture of feces. Some state health departments perform tests to subtype species. In typhoid fever, the organism can be cultured from blood, bone marrow, urine, or feces. Antibody testing has been used for diagnosis when culturing is unavailable or unrevealing.

TREATMENT

Fluid and electrolyte therapy are given as needed. In general, salmonella gastroenteritis is not treated with antibiotics; exceptions are those patients with an increased risk to progress to invasive disease. Those patients include immunocompromised persons, those with chronic inflammatory bowel disease, patients with hemoglobinopathies, those with dysentery, and young infants with a failure-to-thrive syndrome or who are less than 3 months of age. Antibiotic therapy is given for typhoid fever for 2 weeks. Antibiotics that are effective when the organism is susceptible by laboratory testing may include ampicillin (intravenously), amoxicillin, trimethoprim-sulfamethoxazole (intravenously or orally), cefixime, cefotaxime, ceftriaxone, azithromycin, and ciprofloxacin (for adults). Bloodstream and focal infections caused by nontyphoid fever strains of salmonella are treated with the same antibiotics.

INFECTIOUS PERIOD

Asymptomatic individuals with salmonella colonization often excrete the organisms for many months; this is particularly true of children less than 5 years of age. Salmonella infection in daycare centers and preschools has not been a problem, probably because the infectious dose of organisms is high.

INFECTION CONTROL

Parental Advice ► Parents should be advised that spread of salmonella is extremely unlikely in the daycare or preschool setting. If diarrheal symptoms arise, the child should be examined and the stool cultured by his or her health care provider.

Vaccine ▶ The live, attenuated oral vaccine is suitable for administration to children greater than 6 years of age. The Vi capsular polysaccharide vaccine is available for injection in children greater than 2 years of age. Both vaccines are given to family members of a typhoid carrier, selected travelers to areas where the disease is prevalent, persons with continued household contact with a documented typhoid fever carrier, selected laboratory workers, and military personnel.

Exclusion from Daycare or Preschool Attendance ▶ Children should be excluded from daycare or preschool attendance until the diarrhea ceases.

Recommendations for Other Children ▶ There is no action indicated for other children in the daycare or preschool setting once one child is known to be infected. Other children with diarrhea should be seen by their physician.

Recommendations for Personnel ▶ There is no action other than scrupulous handwashing indicated for personnel in the daycare or preschool setting once a child is known to be infected. Staff members diagnosed with *S. typhi* should not work if symptomatic and should not be involved with food preparation until three consecutive stool cultures are negative for *S. typhi*. If more than one case occurs, public health providers should assist in screening food handlers and potentially infected personnel.

58

SCABIES

David A. Whiting

SIGNS AND SYMPTOMS

Scabies causes a severe itch that is usually worse at night. Burrows and vesicles are indicative of mite infestation. Burrows are 5 to 15 millimeters long and often are curved or S-shaped in appearance. They usually occur on wrist flexures, on the ulnar or outer edge of the hand, and in fingerwebs. They also involve the elbows, anterior axillary or elbow folds, nipples, genitalia, and buttocks. Nodular lesions that contain mites sometimes occur, especially on the buttocks and genitalia. Secondary lesions with small papules and scratches and crusts may occur on the abdomen, thighs, and buttocks.

In infants, blisters can occur on the palms and soles. Secondary bacterial infection is common and is usually caused by group A *Streptococcus pyogenes* or *Staphylococcus aureus*. Nodules can be very persistent. Lesions are rare on the scalp and usually only occur in infants.

CAUSE

Scabies is caused by *Sarcoptes scabiei var. hominis*. This is a white, hemispherical mite with four pairs of short legs.

SPREAD AND CONTROL

Source of the Organism ▸ The human body is the only known source of this mite.

High-Risk Populations ▸ Populations at high risk of infection are those in congested housing with overcrowded sleeping quarters. Scabies can be widespread in immunosuppressed individuals or in mentally disabled patients who do not scratch.

Mode of Spread ▸ Spread is from human to human. The mite can only survive up to a few days off the human body, so spread by bedding and clothing is rare.

Incubation Period ▸ The incubation period from egg to adult is 14 to 17 days.

DIAGNOSIS

Definitive diagnosis depends on the microscopic demonstration of a scabies mite from a burrow on the skin. Supporting evidence is provided by an intensely itchy rash affecting the wrists, fingerwebs, elbows, axillary folds, nipples, buttocks, and genitalia, or palms and soles in infants, and by a history of contact with other cases.

TREATMENT

Outpatient therapy is adequate.

The traditional treatment is 1 percent lindane lotion applied from the neck to the toes for 6 to 8 hours. It can be applied to older children and adults for 8 to 12 hours and to small children for a maximum of 6 hours. Due to possible toxicity to the central nervous system, it should not be used in infants, nor in very sick children, nor in children with inflamed and secondarily infected skin. The treatment should not be repeated in less than 7 days, the 1 percent strength of lindane should not be exceeded, and as little as possible should be used. A safer and more effective treatment for all ages is 5 percent permethrin topical cream applied once from head to foot, for 8 to 14 hours. Another safe treatment for small children is 3 to 10 percent sulfur in Eucerin cream applied to the whole body from the neck to the toes for 3 successive nights. Normal laundering of clothes and bedding in a domestic washing machine and dryer is all that is required after treatment.

Ivermectin (an antihelmintic), in a single oral dose has been found to be effective in treating scabies in various parts of the world.

INFECTIOUS PERIOD

The condition is infectious as long as living mites are present on the patient.

INFECTION CONTROL

Parental Advice ▶ Parents and family contacts of an affected child should be treated.

Vaccine ▶ None available.

Exclusion from Daycare or Preschool Attendance ▶ The child should be isolated until effective treatment has been provided.

Recommendations for Other Children ▶ Once one child is infected, it is recommended that all children in the center be treated as though infected.

Recommendations for Personnel ▶ Treatment is recommended for all personnel in the center.

59

SHIGELLA

Linda A. Waggoner-Fountain

SIGNS AND SYMPTOMS

The principal illness caused by shigella is diarrhea. Rare manifestations are bloodstream infection, hemolytic-uremic syndrome, pneumonia, skeletal infections, meningitis, urinary tract infection, and vaginitis.

There are three clinical syndromes of diarrheal disease caused by shigella. The first is the classic bacillary dysentery syndrome manifested by low-grade or moderate fever, cramping abdominal pain, urgent need to defecate, and frequent small-volume stools containing mucus, pus, and sometimes blood. Untreated, it persists for a week or longer.

The second syndrome is the small bowel diarrheal illness. It is characterized by the abrupt onset of high fever, sometimes associated with a seizure; vomiting one or two times; and large-volume, explosive, watery stools. There is spontaneous cure in 24 to 72 hours.

The third syndrome is the small bowel illness just described progressing to dysentery syndrome. During the watery diarrhea phase, one can predict this sequence if white blood cells are seen on microscopic examination of the stool.

CAUSE

Shigella is a gram-negative enteric bacillus whose only natural host is the human. There are four species. *S. flexneri* is most common in developing countries, while *S. sonnei* predominates in developed countries. *S. sonnei* and *S. flexneri* are the two species most likely to be isolated in the United States. *S. dysenteriae* is uncommon but produces severe disease often complicated by hemolytic-uremic syndrome. *S. boydii* is rare.

SPREAD AND CONTROL

Source of the Organism ▶ Humans. There are no animal reservoirs of the shigella organism.

High-Risk Populations ▶ Crowded, unsanitary conditions and lack of refrigeration for food are risk factors. Child daycare populations are a particularly high-risk group. Incidence of disease is also high in institutions for individuals with intellectual and other disabilities. Sexual transmission can occur, especially with oral–anal contact.

Mode of Spread ▶ Spread is from person to person by the fecal–oral route either directly or indirectly through contaminated food or fluids. Shigella organisms are easily spread by direct fecal–oral contact because the number of organisms needed to produce disease is small. A variety of foods have been implicated in the spread of shigella, including salads (potato, tuna, shrimp, macaroni, and chicken), raw vegetables, milk and dairy products, and poultry, as well as common-source water supplies. Rodents, flies, and cockroaches have been implicated in the mechanical transfer of organisms. The chronic carrier state is unusual except in malnourished individuals.

Incubation Period ▶ The interval from ingestion of organisms to onset of symptoms is usually 12 to 48 hours but can be as long as 7 days.

DIAGNOSIS

The diagnosis is generally based on culture of shigella from feces. There are both shigella-specific DNA tests and DNA polymerase chain reaction (PCR) detection tests available, however, these studies are only done in some clinical laboratories. There are no useful antibody tests. A stool smear stained with methylene blue may show white blood cells and an elevated blood fecal lactoferrin, and both are findings consistent with shigella infection.

TREATMENT

Antibiotic therapy of the dysenteric form of illness is effective in shortening the illness and the period of time the patient is infectious to others. Increasing antibiotic resistance is common in shigella organisms, so antibiotic susceptibility testing is important. With significant illness, intravenous or intramuscular ceftriaxone is indicated for therapy. Most isolates in the United States are susceptible to ceftriaxone and ciprofloxacin. Of the antimicrobials available for use in children, trimethoprim-sulfamethoxazole is most commonly used; other drugs effective when the strain is susceptible by laboratory testing are ampicillin, azithromycin, cefixime, tetracycline, nalidixic acid, and fluoroquinolones. The fluoroquinolones are not approved for use in children. Fluid and electrolyte therapy is accomplished with oral rehydration solutions or intravenous fluids. Intestinal antimotility drugs should not be used because they may prolong the clinical and bacteriologic course of disease and eradication of the shigella organism.

INFECTIOUS PERIOD

Shigella cannot be recovered in stool cultures after an average of 2 days following the initiation of antibiotic therapy. Untreated patients usually carry the organism for 7 to 30 days.

INFECTION CONTROL

Parental Advice ▶ Other family members are at risk of becoming infected from children. If diarrhea develops, parents should inform their physician that their child has shigellosis.

Vaccine ▶ There have been many candidate vaccines tested, but no vaccine is available for routine use.

307

Exclusion from Daycare or Preschool Attendance ▶ The child should not attend daycare or preschool until completion of 5 days of antibiotics or until two successive stool cultures are negative or until the diarrhea and systemic symptoms have resolved.

Recommendations for Other Children and Personnel ▶ No action is required for a single case. If there are multiple cases, stool cultures should be obtained on all symptomatic children and personnel to identify and treat infected individuals. Handwashing practices should be reviewed and improved when necessary.

60

STAPHYLOCOCCUS

(Impetigo, Boils, Abscess, Cellulitis, Lymphadenitis, Osteomyelitis, Endocarditis)

Stephanie H. Stovall
Richard F. Jacobs

SIGNS AND SYMPTOMS

Staphylococcal infections (in particular *Staphylococcus aureus*) are commonly associated with diseases of the skin (bullous impetigo, furuncles, or boils), bones and joints (osteomyelitis, septic arthritis), lungs (pneumonia), and heart (endocarditis). Staphylococci cause a wide variety of localized pus-producing diseases but also may cause bloodstream and toxin-mediated diseases (food poisoning, toxic shock syndrome, and staphylococcal scalded skin syndrome). Skin and soft tissue infection is the most common staphylococcal infection of children in day-care centers and preschools. These infections vary in severity from impetigo to furuncles (boils), folliculitis (infection of the hair follicles), cellulitis, or wound infections. Staphylococci are also a frequent cause of lymphadenitis seen most commonly in the neck area in children. Respiratory tract infections, including ear infection, sinusitis, and mastoiditis, have variable involvement by staphylococci, but these organisms can cause severe community-acquired pneumonia or post-viral pneumonia.

Staphylococci are the most common cause of bone and joint infections in children and should be suspected in children with a limp and fever, refusal to walk, and swollen extremities or joints, and in younger children with fever and irritability but no other obvious source of infection. Staphylococcal food poisoning is characterized by the abrupt onset of severe cramps, vomiting, and diarrhea. The short incubation (30 minutes to 7 hours), short duration of illness, epidemiology, and lack of fever help distinguish it from the other causes of food poisoning. Staphylococcal scalded skin syndrome (SSSS) is recognized by peeling of the upper skin layers. Staphylococcal toxic shock syndrome is an acute febrile illness with shock, muscle aches (myalgias), vomiting, diarrhea, sore throat, rash (diffuse sunburn appearance with subsequent peeling), and mucous membrane inflammation.

CAUSE

Staphylococcus aureus is a gram-positive bacterium that grows on most bacteriologic media and produces an enzyme, coagulase, which is important in tissue breakdown and pus formation. The organisms are resistant to heating (up to 122°F), drying, and high salt concentrations, and can survive indefinitely on surfaces, in clothing, and on contaminated objects. Over the last 15 years, community-acquired methicillin-resistant *Staphylococcus aureus* (MRSA) has become an increasing concern. MRSA has become the leading pathogen in skin and soft tissue infection in children. These isolates are usually susceptible to clindamycin and trimethoprim-sulfamethoxazole (TMP-SMX). Resistance and intermediate susceptibility to vancomycin occurs sporadically in patients with extensive contact with healthcare systems and those who have received multiple courses of systemic vancomycin.

SPREAD AND CONTROL

Source of the Organism ▸ Staphylococci are ubiquitous and are found on most environmental surfaces. *Staphylococcus* *aureus* frequently colonizes the skin and mucous membranes of children and adults. Common sites of colonization include: the nose, throat, axilla, hands (transient), and inflamed skin (peeling skin and chronic skin disorders).

High-Risk Populations ▶ Newborns, immunodeficient children, children with recent surgical placement of indwelling devices (intravascular catheters, ventriculoperitoneal shunts) and those with chronic skin conditions such as eczema are high-risk populations. Crowding, poor hygiene, or inadequate infection control measures are predisposing factors.

Mode of Spread ▶ Contact with infected persons, contact with asymptomatic carriers, airborne spread, and contact through contaminated objects all have the potential to spread staphylococci.

Incubation Period ▶ The incubation period is usually 1 to 10 days for skin and soft tissue infections. Other staphylococcal infections may have an incubation period from days to weeks. Toxin-mediated disease typically occurs 1 to 10 days after acquisition, but postoperative toxic shock syndrome may occur within hours.

DIAGNOSIS

Purulent drainage, bullous lesions, or bone and joint infection in a child suggests staphylococcal infection. Microscopic examination of material from lesions with draining pus can provide a presumptive diagnosis. Culture of infected material remains the confirmatory test. Due to recent increases in community-acquired MRSA isolates, susceptibility testing should be done on all isolates. The diagnosis of toxic shock syndrome is made based upon clinical criteria and may have no positive cultures.

TREATMENT

The severity, extent of involvement, organ system involvement, age of the child, and antibiotic susceptibilities dictate the necessity for hospitalization and intravenous antibiotic therapy. For superficial infections, aggressive local care and topical antibiotics may be sufficient. Abscesses should be surgically drained. The mainstay of antistaphylococcal therapy remains antibiotics. The choice of antibiotics must be made after susceptibility tests are available. Most mild to moderate staphylococcal infections can be treated with 7 to 10 days of oral antibiotics. Empiric therapy for mild or moderate staphylococcal infections often includes clindamycin or trimethoprim-sulfa while awaiting susceptibility testing; however, for severe or invasive disease, initial therapy should include vancomycin. The site of infection in serious staphylococcal disease (pneumonia, endocarditis, osteomyelitis) dictates the duration of intravenous therapy. The identification of invasive MRSA or disseminated infection should prompt consultation with a specialist in pediatric infectious diseases as combination therapy, vancomycin therapy, or the use of alternative agents such as linezolid or daptomycin may be indicated.

INFECTIOUS PERIOD

Patients with draining staphylococcal lesions should have lesions covered with a clean, dry dressing. Appropriate hand hygiene by all personnel and children is paramount to prevent spread.

INFECTION CONTROL

Parental Advice ▶ Parents should institute close observation for early signs of staphylococcal infection with prompt recognition and treatment. Any child with clinical evidence of staphylococcal disease should be taken to their local pediatrician for diagnosis and therapy.

Vaccine ▶ None available.

Exclusion from Daycare or Preschool Attendance ▶ The child with a draining staphylococcal infection must have the lesion covered with a clean and dry dressing during daycare or preschool attendance. If this is impossible, the child should be excluded until the wound is improved.

Recommendations for Other Children ▶ The best recommendation is prevention of spread. This includes proper disinfection procedures, good handwashing, avoidance of open infected wounds, improved hygiene, and reduced crowding. Children with suspected staphylococcal infection should be referred to their pediatrician. In situations of multiple cases (outbreak), all infected children should be referred to their pediatrician, and consideration of temporary closure of the facility should be discussed with local experts and public health officials until the infections are controlled. In a MRSA outbreak, grouping of possibly infected children, and good handwashing, are critical.

Recommendations for Personnel ▶ The involved personnel should implement contact isolation, improved handwashing, and early recognition and treatment of infected children. No routine cultures or antibiotic therapy (oral or topical) is indicated for contacts unless an epidemic occurs.

61

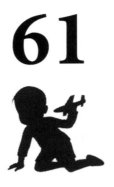

STREPTOCOCCUS

(Cellulitis, Impetigo, Pharyngitis)

Stephanie H. Stovall
Richard F. Jacobs

SIGNS AND SYMPTOMS

The most common illnesses associated with group A beta hemolytic streptococci (GABHS) are sore throat (pharyngitis) and impetigo. Sore throat varies greatly in severity from subclinical to severe, with high fever, nausea, vomiting, and collapse. The onset is usually acute, with sore throat, fever, headache, and/or abdominal pain. The throat and tonsils usually appear red and swollen with pus on the tonsils in 50 to 90 percent of patients and a rash on the palate. Pus on the tonsils usually appears around day 2, is whitish-yellow, and appears early as discrete spots that then progress to one large patch. Swollen, tender lymph nodes in the neck are found in 40 to 60 percent of cases. Clinical manifestations usually subside spontaneously in 3 to 5 days unless complications (peritonsillar abscess) occur. An infantile form (children less than 3 years of age) may occur with GABHS and is more prolonged with persistent purulent nasal discharge, fever, and lymphadenopathy. Non-infectious complications may occur in approximately 10 days (nephritis) to 18 days (acute rheumatic fever). Scarlet fever represents another unusual manifestation of GABHS, with a red raised rash on the trunk that spreads to the arms and legs within several hours to days. When this rash does occur, it has a typical "sandpaper" feel, fades on pressure, and usually peels. The rash may have a non-blanching component in the joint folds (Pastia's lines), and is often associated with a strawberry tongue and red swollen lips. Scarlet fever occurs commonly with pharyngitis, but may also occur with streptococcal skin infection.

Impetigo is the the most common skin manifestation of GABHS. Impetigo lesions most commonly occur over scratched areas, such as insect bites, where the germ is introduced into normal skin. The skin lesions usually start as superficial vesicles or red pustules and progress to thick yellowish crusted lesions that last from days to several weeks. Fever or constitutional symptoms rarely accompany impetigo. A whole body diffuse rash (scarlatiniform) may accompany impetigo lesions. Secondary infection with staphylococci is common and may lead to pustules or cellulitis. This type of superficial infected rash may complicate abnormal skin (eczema) or follow trauma or burns. Glomerulonephritis is the most common non-infectious complication and usually occurs around 3 weeks after the skin infection.

Other infections associated with GABHS include more serious skin infections (cellulitis, erysipelas), ear infection, sinusitis, pneumonia, perianal cellulitis, vaginitis, and invasive disease (streptococcal toxic shock syndrome and necrotizing fasciitis which usually follows varicella-zoster virus [VZV] infection).

CAUSE

GABHS are gram-positive cocci. More than 80 different types of GABHS are known.

SPREAD AND CONTROL

Source of the Organism ▶ Upper respiratory tract and skin lesions are the most common source of GABHS. Cases of invasive GABHS disease in close contacts of patients with invasive disease have been reported. Contaminated food or milk has caused some outbreaks, and anal carriage has been linked to several hospital outbreaks. Recent evidence indicates that children in daycare centers are colonized with GABHS at an earlier age. Reports of several outbreaks of GABHS in daycare centers have been published.

High-Risk Populations ► Crowding, poor hygiene, and improper handling of infected children are associated with the greatest risk of transmission and predisposition to GABHS disease. Children less than 3 years of age are less likely to have GABHS pharyngitis. Children with diagnosed acute rheumatic fever are a high-risk population for acquisition and recurrences. Children with varicella-zoster virus infection are predisposed to invasive GABHS disease.

Mode of Spread ► Close contact with an infected individual by direct projection of large respiratory droplets (not aerosols) or physical transfer of respiratory secretions or infected skin lesions.

Incubation Period ► Streptococcal pharyngitis: 12 hours to 4 days. Streptococcal impetigo: few days to several weeks (usually around 10 days). Invasive GABHS disease: few days to a week (case reports). Toxic shock syndrome can occur within hours of inoculation.

DIAGNOSIS

The clinical appearance and epidemiology should provide the caretaker with a high degree of suspicion. Culture of the tonsils or infected skin lesions with the isolation of GABHS is diagnostic. Due to the time frame for this procedure, a number of rapid detection kits for identifying GABHS pharyngitis in minutes to hours have been developed. If the rapid test is negative, a culture should be obtained to confirm a negative rapid test. Positive results from rapid antigen tests or throat cultures do not distinguish GABHS carriage from acute GABHS infection. Epidemiologic factors and clinical symptoms and signs should be used to determine the need for GABHS testing to avoid unnecessary treatment in children who may have viral pharyngitis and are only colonized with GABHS.

TREATMENT

The therapy for GABHS pharyngitis is antibiotics; penicillin is the drug of choice. It is usually given as a single intramuscular injection of long-acting penicillin or oral penicillin for 10 full days. Amoxicillin suspension is often preferred to penicillin suspension because it tastes better. Either a narrow spectrum cephalosporin or clindamycin are appropriate or effective choices for patients with a history of allergy to penicillins. Most treatment failures likely result from failure to take the antibiotic for the full course as opposed to bacteriologic failure. For GABHS impetigo, local care with abrasive cleansing of lesions is effective. Oral penicillin or an antistaphylococcal antibiotic may be beneficial in children with numerous lesions. Hospitalization is only required for invasive disease. The current recommendation for treatment of invasive GABHS disease is the combination of penicillin plus clindamycin.

INFECTIOUS PERIOD

The period of maximal infectivity is in the acute phase of the illness with most secondary cases occurring within 2 weeks of acquisition.

INFECTION CONTROL

Parental Advice ▶ If the child becomes symptomatic, he or she should be taken to the local pediatrician for diagnostic testing and treatment if positive. If the child has a previous diagnosis of acute rheumatic fever and a history of close contact with a proven GABHS patient, he or she should be taken to the local pediatrician for culture and initiation of prophylactic antibiotics to prevent recurrences of rheumatic fever. Children should be immunized with VZV and influenza vaccines.

Vaccine ▶ None available. However, immunization with VZV vaccine can reduce the risk of varicella-associated invasive GABHS skin disease. Influenza vaccine can reduce the risk of influenza-associated GABHS complications.

Exclusion from Daycare or Preschool Attendance ▶ Infected children should avoid close contact with other children until at least 24 hours after appropriate therapy is started.

Recommendations for Other Children ▶ The best current control measure is prompt recognition and treatment of GABHS infections. The best current control measure for invasive GABHS disease is immunization with VZV and influenza vaccines.

Contacts with recent or current clinical evidence of GABHS infection should be cultured and treated if culture-positive to reduce transmission and nonsuppurative complications. Siblings do have a higher acquisition rate (up to 50 percent).

No data are available to allow for a recommendation about the usefulness of throat cultures or antigen detection tests in identifying contacts at increased risk for invasive GABHS disease. Because the risk of streptococcal infection in contacts is low, chemoprophylaxis is not routinely recommended in families, schools, or childcare facilities. However, some experts have encouraged consideration of chemoprophylaxis for persons with other risk factors for severe GABHS disease (e.g., human immunodeficiency virus, over 65 years of age, or diabetes mellitus) who are or have been in close contact with patients with severe invasive GABHS disease. Many therapeutic regimens have been studied for eradication of GABHS in patients who are chronic carriers. Of the many options, the simplest and most effective is clindamycin.

Recommendations for Personnel ▶ In non-epidemic situations, only symptomatic personnel should be cultured and treated if positive. Screening asymptomatic children or personnel, especially in nonepidemic situations, is not warranted. In epidemics or in family situations in which a child has acute rheumatic fever, selective cultures of contacts may be warranted.

62

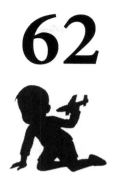

SYPHILIS

(Treponema pallidum)

Michael F. Rein

SIGNS AND SYMPTOMS

Syphilis is an extremely variable and complex disease. It may be encountered in two forms in the daycare center or pre-school: congenital (infected in utero) or acquired (infected at or after delivery). Early congenital syphilis usually manifests during the first 3 months of life and includes a generalized rash, which may appear blister-like and often involves the palms and soles, although it is frequently confined to the diaper area. Syphilis may also cause enlargement of the liver or spleen, enlargement of lymph nodes, or meningitis. Of particular public health importance are "snuffles," a chronic nasal discharge, and mucous patches, which are painless ulcers inside the mouth. Both contain large numbers of organisms and are highly contagious. Warty lesions, called condylomata lata, may develop around the anus or vagina. Late congenital syphilis is not contagious and presents with a variety of skeletal lesions, including frontal enlargement of the skull, anterior curving of the shins, collapse of the nose, or notching of the secondary incisors (front teeth). One may also see inflammation of the corneas, called interstitial keratitis, which usually appears between the ages of 5 and 16 years; and mild to moderate deafness.

Acquired syphilis results from contact, usually sexual, with an infected lesion. Infected patients develop a painless lesion, called a chancre, at the point of inoculation, the exact site of which depends on the practice that resulted in infection (e.g., around the mouth or anus). Secondary syphilis occurs weeks to months later and consists initially of a nonspecific febrile illness followed by a generalized, relatively indolent rash and generalized swelling of lymph nodes. There may be patchy hair loss and mucous patches. The dry skin lesions are not contagious, but the mucous patches contain large numbers of organisms and can spread infection. Secondary syphilis may also present as liver or kidney disease. Primary and secondary syphilis resolve without specific treatment, but the patient remains infected. Antibiotic therapy given for other infections may modify or completely mask the clinical manifestations of syphilis.

CAUSE

Treponema pallidum is a spirochete that does not survive in the environment. It can penetrate mucous membranes and even intact-appearing skin, and it remains highly sensitive to many antibiotics.

SPREAD AND CONTROL

Source of the Organism ► The fetus can be infected by spirochetes passing through the placenta from the maternal bloodstream. Newborns may also acquire the organism from mothers during delivery. In older children, acquisition is almost exclusively sexual.

High-Risk Populations ► Syphilis in pregnant women, and hence congenital syphilis, is usually associated with maternal youth, poverty, and psychosocial problems. Older children with syphilis tend to come from similar backgrounds, and/or have been sexually abused by infected persons.

Mode of Spread ▸ Acquisition of the organism after birth requires direct contact with infectious material. Thus, older children with acquired syphilis must be evaluated for sexual abuse. However, the organism may also be transmitted in blood and by some of the lesions of secondary syphilis, such as mucous patches of the mouth.

Incubation Period ▸ The incubation period of acquired syphilis is usually 10 to 21 days but may extend to 90 days.

DIAGNOSIS

Syphilis is subclinical (invisible) during much of its course, and thus diagnosis usually depends on testing the blood for antibodies to *T. pallidum* using any of a variety of newly developed tests. A positive test is followed by one of the older types of tests (e.g., RPR, VDRL), which can then be used to assess the adequacy of treatment. Diagnosis in the newborn is more complicated, because maternal antibody acquired transplacentally may obscure the infant's immune response for several months. Organisms in chancres, condylomata lata, mucous patches, and the infected nasal secretions of newborns may be detected with special laboratory techniques.

TREATMENT

Various forms of penicillin remain effective treatment for congenital or acquired syphilis. Infants with congenital syphilis require either procaine penicillin given intramuscularly once daily or aqueous crystalline penicillin G given intravenously for 10 days. Hospitalization is usually required for the treatment of congenital syphilis and may also be indicated for management of sexually abused children. Children more than one month of age with acquired syphilis, and some children with a normal physical examination but at risk for congenital syphilis, may be treated with a single administration of intramuscular benzathine penicillin G. It is essential that Bicillin® L-A and not Bicillin® C-R be used for this purpose. The treatment of persons allergic to penicillin is complex and should be undertaken in consultation with an expert.

Congenital syphilis should be considered a "sentinel health event" that indicates a breakdown of health care for the family.

Acquired syphilis must be evaluated as sexual abuse. Children with syphilis should be evaluated for other sexually transmitted infections, including infection with the human immunodeficiency virus (HIV).

INFECTIOUS PERIOD

The infected person is no longer contagious 24 hours after receiving effective treatment. Without therapy, the period of contagiousness may last for months.

INFECTION CONTROL

Parental Advice ▶ If the infection was not acquired at the daycare center or preschool, other parents should not be informed, because the infection is stigmatizing, and the risk of transmission is extremely low. Detection of the infection may have forensic implications for the daycare center or preschool.

Vaccine ▶ None available.

Exclusion from Daycare or Preschool Attendance ▶ The child may return to daycare the day after being given effective treatment.

Recommendations for Other Children ▶ The risk of non-sexual transmission to other children is low, but real. If the child acquired infection elsewhere and has been treated, no further measures for control of infection are necessary. The child, however, may be at risk of emotional and behavioral problems.

Recommendations for Personnel ▶ Careful handwashing and the use of antibacterial gels and lotions are essential. The risk of transmission to personnel is low, but real.

63

TINEA CAPITIS, CORPORIS, CRURIS, AND PEDIS

(Ringworm, Athlete's Foot, Jock Itch)

David A. Whiting

SIGNS AND SYMPTOMS

Tinea capitis (head): This condition causes partial hair loss. Patches vary from well-circumscribed, round lesions to vague and irregular areas of hair thinning that are difficult to detect. Redness and scaling may be present and can range from mild to severe. In the United States, affected hairs are generally broken off flush with the scalp and appear as black dots when due to infection by *Trichophyton tonsurans*, but occasionally are grayish-white and are broken off 1 to 3 mm above the skin surface when due to *Microsporum canis* infection. Inflammatory types of scalp ringworm sometimes cause fluctuant, boggy, purulent masses associated with hair loss, a so-called kerion infection. The incidence of tinea capitis is equal in males and females. Tinea capitis peaks at age 5 and usually disappears at puberty, although there are specific types that can affect adults.

Tinea corporis (body): This condition usually starts as small, reddish, itchy, scaly dots that gradually expand outward, clearing in the middle, forming annular lesions with scaly margins and clear centers. Sometimes, new lesions form in the middle of an expanding lesion and spread outward to cause concentric rings. The lesions are usually single but, if multiple, are often unilateral or at least asymmetrical.

Tinea cruris (groin): This condition is rare before puberty. It causes itchy, reddish, and scaly lesions in the groin and on the adjacent thighs, and may extend around the anus onto the buttocks, with advancing scaly borders and central clearing. Some types of tinea cruris, especially those due to *Trichophyton rubrum*, may produce large, circular lesions around the genitalia.

Tinea pedis (foot): This condition is also rare before puberty. There are three types; namely, the interdigital, the vesicular, and the moccasin. The interdigital type usually starts in the lateral toe webs and spreads medially, and the vesicular type generally affects the instep. The lesions are usually unilateral and asymmetrical, except for the moccasin type of tinea pedis in which both feet are affected by a diffuse, scaling rash. Tinea pedis is aggravated by heat and sweating.

CAUSE

Tinea infections are caused by one or more of the dermatophytes, or skin fungi. Infection is confined to keratin, the dead horn of skin, hair, and nails. At present, 39 different species of dermatophytes are recognized in humans and almost all human infections are caused by 16 species, only 5 of which are common in the United States.

SPREAD AND CONTROL

Source of the Organism ▶ Human source: *Trichophyton tonsurans, Microsporum audouinii, T. rubrum,* and *Epidermophyton floccosum.* Animal source: *M. canis, T. mentagrophytes,* and *T. verrucosum.* Soil source: *M. gypseum.*

High-Risk Populations ▶ Children aged 2 to 20 years are at the greatest risk. Overcrowding with head-to-head contact predisposes to ringworm of the scalp. Contact with cattle and horses can result in animal ringworm.

Mode of Spread ▸ Tinea is spread by direct contact with humans, animals, or soil or by indirect contact with contaminated combs, brushes, headgear, towels, pillows, bedding, or clothing.

Incubation Period ▸ It takes 3 to 5 days for microscopic infection and 2 to 3 weeks for clinical manifestations to develop. The condition can spread for 3 to 4 months, and then, after a refractory period, spontaneous regression may occur.

DIAGNOSIS

The diagnosis is made on the clinical appearance; positive Wood's light examination in some cases of tinea capitis; microscopic demonstration of the fungus in potassium hydroxide preparations of skin, hair, and nails; and fungal culture.

TREATMENT

All treatment is managed on an outpatient basis.

Tinea capitis (head): The preferred treatment is griseofulvin taken orally for 6 to 12 weeks. Second-choice therapy is ketoconazole for 6 to 12 weeks. Oral itraconazole, fluconazole, and terbinafine are other effective therapies. To prevent cross infection, clip the affected hairs and shampoo with selenium sulfide (2.5 percent) twice weekly or apply a topical antifungal preparation, as for tinea corporis, daily.

Tinea corporis (body): Topical clotrimazole, econazole, ketoconazole, miconazole nitrate, oxiconazole, sulconazole, naftifine, butenafine, terbinafine, or ciclopirox olamine can be used once or twice daily. A salicylic acid and benzoic acid combination can be used. In severe cases, oral griseofulvin, terbinafine, or itraconazole is recommended.

Tinea pedis (foot): In the inflammatory stage, soaks with Burow's solution or potassium permanganate solution can be used. The fungal infection can be treated topically as for tinea corporis, and undecylenate powder can be sprinkled in the socks. Oral griseofulvin, itraconazole, or terbinafine may be necessary (see above).

Tinea cruris (groin): Topical antifungal therapy as for tinea corporis. In addition, oral griseofulvin or terbinafine may be necessary in extensive cases.

INFECTIOUS PERIOD

The patient is infectious as long as organisms can be found invading the tissue on microscopic examination or by culture. Tinea capitis may persist from 3 months to several years. Tinea corporis may persist or recur for many years, as may tinea cruris or tinea pedis.

INFECTION CONTROL

Parental Advice ▶ Parents should be notified that there has been a case or cases of tinea in the center. They should watch for the development of infection and seek medical attention for diagnosis and therapy as necessary.

Vaccine ▶ None available.

Exclusion from Daycare or Preschool Attendance ▶ No isolation needed after effective treatment is started.

Recommendations for Other Children ▶ Watch for development of infection and treat if necessary.

Recommendations for Personnel ▶ Watch for development of infection and treat if necessary.

64

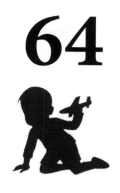

TOXOCARA

Jonathan P. Moorman

SIGNS AND SYMPTOMS

The clinical manifestations of toxocara infection depend on the size of the infecting dose of larvae. Individuals who ingest small numbers of larvae may remain without symptoms, while those ingesting large numbers may develop a disseminated infection called visceral larva migrans. Characteristic findings in visceral larva migrans include fever, liver enlargement, eosinophilia, and hypergammaglobulinemia. A cough, wheezing, and pulmonary infiltrates may also be present, and, rarely, heart inflammation and neurologic inflammation may develop. Toxocara larvae may invade the eye, producing retinal lesions or inflammation and occasionally resulting in blindness. Ocular larva migrans is not characterized by hepatomegaly and eosinophilia, and visceral and ocular larva migrans are rarely observed concurrently.

CAUSE

Toxocariasis is caused by *Toxocara canis* and *Toxocara cati*, common roundworms of dogs and cats; the majority of cases in this country are due to *T. canis*. Dogs and cats are commonly infected by Toxocara, with most having acquired the infection early in life. Infected animals harbor adult worms that pass eggs in the feces. After several weeks in soil, infective larvae develop within the eggs. Humans acquire toxocariasis by ingesting eggs that then hatch in the small intestine, releasing the larvae. After penetrating the intestinal wall, the larvae begin to migrate throughout human host tissues. The larvae cannot complete their normal development in humans, and therefore they do not mature into adult worms capable of passing eggs in human feces. After a variable period of migration, the larvae within a human host will eventually die.

SPREAD AND CONTROL

Source of the Organism ▸ Toxocara infections occur in both temperate and tropical areas, being most prevalent where dogs are common and hygiene is poor. Eggs passed in dog and cat feces become infective after approximately 3 weeks in the soil and may persist in the environment for months. Parks and playgrounds are often heavily contaminated, providing a ready source of infective eggs. Ingestion of even small amounts of dirt may result in the transmission of relatively large numbers of eggs.

High-Risk Populations ▸ Children less than 6 years of age are at higher risk of acquiring toxocariasis because they are more likely to eat dirt and to contaminate their hands and food.

Mode of Spread ▸ Humans acquire toxocara infections by ingesting soil containing infective eggs. Transmission is generally the result of eating dirt in young children and of exposure to hands or possibly food contaminated with infective eggs in older children. As humans do not pass Toxocara eggs in their feces, person-to-person transmission of the infection does not occur.

Incubation Period ▸ The time interval between acquisition of infection and the development of visceral larva migrans appears to be quite variable, ranging from days to months. Although not well established, the incubation period prior to the development of ocular larva migrans appears to be longer, ranging from months to years.

DIAGNOSIS

Visceral larva migrans should be considered in any child with a history of eating dirt or exposure to dogs who presents with blood testing that reveals high eosinophil numbers and gammaglobulin levels. Elevated titers of isohemagglutinins to the A and B blood group antigens are also often present in toxocariasis. The diagnosis can be confirmed by demonstration of larvae in a liver biopsy; however, the larvae may be difficult to find, and a negative liver biopsy does not rule out the diagnosis. A specific antibody test, available at the Centers for Disease Control and Prevention, can be used to establish a serologic diagnosis.

TREATMENT

To date, no studies have proved the effectiveness of any therapeutic regimen against toxocariasis. Mebendazole and albendazole have been used to treat toxocariasis and appear to be associated with few adverse effects. These drugs are considered investigational for this condition by the FDA. Treatment with diethylcarbamazine has been reported to decrease symptoms in some patients. Corticosteroids have also been used in individuals with significant involvement of the heart or central nervous system. Optimal therapy for ocular larva migrans has not been well established; past approaches have included the use of antihelmintic agents and corticosteroids.

INFECTIOUS PERIOD

Humans with toxocariasis are not infectious.

INFECTION CONTROL

Parental Advice ▶ Parents should be reassured that a child with toxocariasis will not transmit the infection to other children. The mode of spread should be explained to them, emphasizing the need to keep their children from eating dirt and to properly dispose of cat and dog feces. Pet owners should be encouraged to seek expert advice from a veterinarian regarding treatment of puppies and kittens with appropriate antihelmintics to avoid exposing their children to toxocara. In addition, dogs and especially puppies should be periodically examined for the presence of helminths.

Vaccine ► None available.

Exclusion from Daycare or Preschool Attendance ► A child with toxocariasis cannot transmit the infection to other individuals and therefore does not need to be kept out of any daycare or preschool setting.

Recommendations for Other Children ► Other children in the center will acquire toxocariasis only if they ingest soil containing infective eggs. Given the high prevalence of infective eggs in most communities, children should not be allowed to eat dirt, and good hygiene should be enforced.

Recommendations for Personnel ► Personnel should minimize their exposure to infective toxocara eggs by maintaining good hygienic practices. They should also attempt to diminish children's exposure by not letting them eat dirt and by covering play areas such as sandboxes in order to prevent animals from defecating in them.

65

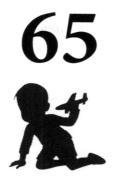

TRICHURIS TRICHIURA

(Whipworm)

Jonathan P. Moorman

SIGNS AND SYMPTOMS

The clinical manifestations associated with *Trichuris trichiura* infections depend on the intensity and duration of the infection and on the age of the host. Light infections are generally asymptomatic. Heavy infections, most often seen in young children, may be associated with malnutrition, mild anemia, diffuse inflammation of the bowel, chronic diarrhea, and rectal prolapse. Stunted growth of children can occur with even moderate infections.

CAUSE

T. trichiura is an intestinal worm also known as the human whipworm. Humans acquire trichuriasis by ingesting infective-stage eggs derived from human feces. The eggs hatch in the small intestine, and the larvae mature into adult worms and attach to the superficial mucosa of the cecum and ascending colon, where they can survive for 5 years. Female worms produce eggs that are passed in the feces; if exposed to favorable conditions of soil, moisture, and temperature, the eggs embryonate, developing into infective-stage ova within 11 to 30 days. Eggs that have not embryonated are not infective.

SPREAD AND CONTROL

Source of the Organism ▸ Although *T. trichiura* infections are found worldwide, they are most prevalent in the tropics, particularly in overcrowded communities with poor sanitation. Infective-stage eggs are found in soil contaminated with human feces, and infection may result from direct ingestion of soil or indirectly through contaminated hands, utensils, or food.

High-Risk Populations ▸ In areas where *T. trichiura* is endemic, children are often infected by the time they are 2 years old, and reinfection is common. Infection of young children is often a consequence of eating dirt, whereas older children and adults are more likely to be infected through indirect contamination by flies and insects.

Mode of Spread ▸ Transmission occurs through the ingestion of infective eggs. As *T. trichiura* eggs are not infective until after they have embryonated in the soil, person-to-person transmission of the infection does not occur.

Incubation Period ▸ The interval between the acquisition of *T. trichiura* and the passage of eggs in the feces is approximately 30 to 90 days. The time from infection to the development of symptoms has not been well established.

DIAGNOSIS

The diagnosis can be made fairly easily by microscopic stool examination with detection of the characteristic eggs. In symptomatic individuals, it may be important to quantitate the intensity of the worm burden, as significant symptoms are rarely associated with light *T. trichiura* infections and may indicate the presence of other pathogenic processes. Adult worms may be seen on direct examination of the rectum and anus or during rectal prolapse in heavy infections. Eosinophilia is rare.

TREATMENT

In countries where trichuriasis is endemic and where reinfection is common, light infections are often untreated. However, in this country, *T. trichiura* infections are generally treated with oral mebendazole. Although mebendazole appears to be somewhat effective and has low toxicity in children, data regarding its use in children younger than 2 years is limited. Ivermectin and albendazole are alternative regimens but are not FDA-approved for this indication.

INFECTIOUS PERIOD

If untreated, trichuriasis may persist for many years.

INFECTION CONTROL

Parental Advice ▶ The mode of spread should be explained to parents, reassuring them that person-to-person transmission does not occur. In *T. trichiura* endemic areas, the need to discourage eating of dirt among young children and to encourage good hygiene among older children should be emphasized to parents.

Vaccine ▶ None available.

Exclusion from Daycare or Preschool Attendance ▶ Children with trichuriasis do not need to be isolated or kept out of any childcare setting. Human-to-human transmission does not appear to occur, and *T. trichiura* eggs are not immediately infectious when passed in feces.

Recommendations for Other Children ▶ Other children in the center will become infected with *T. trichiura* only if they ingest eggs that have embryonated after several weeks in the soil. If fecal contamination of the environment is a problem in the center, children must be kept from ingesting infected dirt either directly or indirectly through contaminated hands or food.

Recommendations for Personnel ▶ Inadvertent contamination of food, utensils, and hands with soil containing infective eggs should be avoided. Personnel should maintain good handwashing practices and ensure the appropriate disposal of fecal material.

66

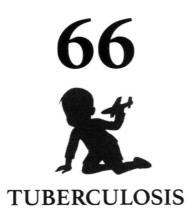

TUBERCULOSIS

Tania A. Thomas

SIGNS AND SYMPTOMS

There is a wide range of manifestations of tuberculosis (TB), from asymptomatic "latent" infection to severe disseminated forms of disease. After exposure to TB, the body works to control the infection resulting in a relative dormant state of infection termed "latent tuberculosis." However, for some, the immune system is unable to control the infection resulting in active, symptomatic disease which may develop as early as a few weeks or as late as a few decades after initial infection. Symptoms typically include cough, fevers, poor appetite, weight loss, decreased energy, and occasionally night sweats. Depending on the age of the child, some symptoms may be subtle or absent.

Overall, only about 5 to 10 percent of children over 2 years of age with latent TB will ever become ill with active disease. Children under 2 years of age are at higher risk of developing active TB after infection. Approximately 50 percent of children infected with TB under the age of 1 year will progress to active disease. Approximately 25 percent of children infected with TB between the ages of 1 and 2 years will progress to active disease. Not only are younger children at increased risk of disease progression, but they tend to develop symptoms more quickly after infection and tend to have more disseminated disease, including meningitis.

Pulmonary disease is the most common manifestation of TB infection. Children with primary pulmonary TB have fever, cough, poor appetite, weight loss, and occasionally wheezing. Examination of these children occasionally may reveal abnormal sounds on lung examination including rales (crackles) and wheezing. Chest X-rays from children most commonly reveal enlarged lymph nodes in the lung regions, but also may reveal lung infiltrates or pneumonia. Adolescents and adults may have cavitary lesions (abscesses) in the lung and more extensive pneumonia seen on chest X-ray, but this is less commonly found in younger children. Similarly, the classic description described in adults of a wet cough or blood-tinged sputum is much rarer in young children.

Infection of the lymph nodes in the neck (scrofula) is another early form of disease caused by *Mycobacterium tuberculosis*. This typically presents with painless, superficial swelling of the lymph nodes in the neck region. Examination reveals enlarged glands that are not warm to touch. Over time, lymph nodes can cluster and occasionally may drain purulent material.

Less frequently, the mycobacteria may spread from the original site of infection in the lungs through the lymphatic system and bloodstream to other organs and cause "extrapulmonary" tuberculosis. The clinical picture that results is determined by the child's age at the time of infection, his/her susceptibility, and the infecting dose. The most serious complications of TB are miliary disease and meningitis, both of which occur within months following the initial infection. Miliary disease refers to disseminated disease commonly with multiorgan involvement. The onset may be insidious or abrupt. The chest X-ray demonstrates a classic pattern of small, uniform lesions resembling millet seeds that are studded throughout both lung fields. Meningitis develops in approximately 2 percent of TB cases, with an increased risk for children less than 5 years of age. There is a high case fatality rate, and many serious neurologic complications occur in the survivors if TB meningitis is not recognized and treated early. The case fatality rate increases with the more advanced stages of disease at the time of diagnosis and initiation of antituberculous therapy.

Other sites of disease include the bones and joints, most notably the spine (Pott's disease) which typically occurs at least 1 to 2 years after initial infection. Sites that are much less commonly affected include the throat, abdomen, kidneys, genital tract, ears, eyes, and skin. Delayed recognition and treatment of these later complications may lead to chronic failure to gain weight and physical deformities. These more extensive types of disease can be prevented by treatment of asymptomatic tuberculous infection or early pulmonary disease.

CAUSE

The agent that causes TB is *Mycobacterium tuberculosis*, often referred to as "M. TB" or the "tubercle bacillus." This mycobacterium is identified presumptively during microscopic examination of body fluids that have been stained with special dyes by its "acid-fast" character and appearance as a red rod. This organism is slow growing and requires up to 6 weeks of incubation on traditional culture media before it can be isolated and the diagnosis confirmed. Automated systems (e.g., BACTEC) may allow isolation after only 1 to 2 weeks of incubation. After the organism is isolated, further biochemical or molecular tests are required to confirm the species, as *M. tuberculosis* shares similarities to other mycobacterial species. Isolation of the infecting organism is critical to allow drug testing that defines which antibiotics are effective. Over the past few decades, antibiotic resistance has developed to the commonly used anti-TB medications. Drug-resistant strains have been classified as multidrug-resistant (MDR) TB and extensively drug-resistant (XDR) TB, based on resistance to the two most potent first-line medications and additional resistance to second-line medications, respectively. Although drug-resistant forms of TB are more commonly encountered in developing countries, they are found in the United States, accounting for less than 5 percent of all cases nationwide.

SPREAD AND CONTROL

Source of the Organism ▸ Adults or adolescents with TB and active respiratory symptoms are the main source of *M.*

tuberculosis for children. Although *Mycobacterium bovis* may cause disease in animals (especially cows), it very rarely causes infection and illness in humans in the United States unless raw milk or cheese from an infected animal are consumed. This distinction is important because *M. bovis* is resistant to pyrazinamide, a drug commonly used to treat *M. tuberculosis*. Dogs are susceptible to the human type of tubercle bacillus, but there is little evidence to support a role for dogs in the transmission of tuberculous infection to children.

High-Risk Populations ► High-risk groups can be divided into those with a high prevalence of TB infection and those who are at increased risk of progressing to active disease once infected.

Populations with a higher prevalence of TB infection include:

- people born in TB-endemic countries;
- people who have lived in or travelled frequently to TB-endemic countries;
- people who are homeless;
- residents and employees of congregate settings including correctional facilities, homeless shelters, and long-term health care facilities;
- healthcare workers; and
- infants and children who are exposed to adults in the above-mentioned high risk settings.

Populations at increased risk of progressing to active TB once infected include:

- people at the extremes of the age spectrum (under 5 years and over 65 years of age);
- people who have been exposed recently (in the past 2 years); and
- people with abnormal immune systems (either due to a primary medical condition or the related treatment) including HIV infection, cancers, organ transplantation, certain rheumatologic conditions, and their immune-suppressing treatments, prolonged steroids, as well as diabetes, chronic kidney failure, silicosis, active substance abuse, and malnutrition.

The most important risk factor for the development of active tuberculosis is the presence of HIV infection and acquired immunodeficiency syndrome (AIDS). There is a nearly 200-fold increase in the risk of active disease in patients with advanced AIDS; the two infections stimulate progression of each other, thus contributing to significant illness and death worldwide.

Tuberculosis can be difficult to diagnose accurately and requires prolonged treatment. Due to the public health infrastructure and resources required for adequate control of this disease, many resource-limited countries still have a high burden of TB. Because of this higher prevalence abroad, certain foreign-born individuals who come from TB-endemic regions may be at higher risk of having latent or active forms of TB.

Children younger than 5 years of age and especially infants in the first year of life have a reduced ability to limit spread of the initial tuberculous infection to other organs. Hormonal changes associated with puberty result in poor healing of the primary focus of infection, and waning immunity of the elderly who have been infected years previously accounts for their characteristic patterns of slowly progressive disease with classic pulmonary abscesses (cavitary lesions).

Mode of Spread ▸ *M. tuberculosis* is transmitted primarily by inhalation of droplet nuclei. The risk factors most highly associated with transmission of infection include:

- high infective dose, commonly associated with untreated adults or adolescents who are actively coughing, not using "cough hygiene" (covering mouth/nose), and have severe disease marked by "smear positivity" (organisms detected in sputum by microscopy alone), extensive pulmonary involvement with or without a cavitary lesion;
- aerosolization of infected body fluids;
- prolonged duration and proximity of exposure; and
- inadequate ventilation system of buildings.

Although repeated direct exposure to infected individuals is usually necessary, it has been shown that sharing a common air supply with a highly infective individual may be sufficient. Once an adult has been confirmed to have active pulmonary TB disease, he/she has already infected, on average, 8 to 15 individuals; however this is highly dependent upon the contagiousness of the patient. Some people who readily have *M. tuberculosis* identified in their sputum samples by microscopic analysis are more infectious, while others are less so. People with latent TB infection are, by definition, without disease and not contagious. Additionally, infants and young children are not commonly considered to be infectious because they typically do not have the ability to cough forcefully enough to aerosolize the infection and the burden of organisms in childhood TB is less than that among adults and adolescents. People who have been on appropriate treatment and have symptom resolution are thought not to be infectious.

People with only "extrapulmonary" forms of TB are not considered infectious. The rare exception may include patients with mycobacterial organisms present in purulent material draining from an infected lymph node, ear, bone, or skin lesions. This material could be infectious to others by direct contact, via hand carriage of a caretaker, or potentially by aerosolization of organisms from the drainage, for example during a wound irrigation procedure. While many outbreaks have occurred in correctional facilities and hospitals, others have been reported within schools and childcare centers. In nearly all of these cases, transmission started with an infectious adult or adolescent, including a child's family member, teacher, or other school staff member. Younger children and infants are rarely able to transmit TB, in contrast to other infections like diarrhea and viral respiratory infections.

Incubation Period ▶ The incubation period from the time the mycobacteria enter the body to the time that the individual develops a positive tuberculin skin test (TST or cutaneous hypersensitivity) may vary from 2 to 10 weeks. The onset of tuberculin hypersensitivity may be accompanied by fever lasting for 1 to 3 weeks. Symptomatic disease may develop within a few weeks of the initial infection (especially for infants) or many years later when the body's normal immune system becomes suppressed either by another disease process or by chemotherapeutic agents used to treat the disease (e.g., human immunodeficiency virus [HIV] infection, diabetes, leukemia, tumors, bone marrow, or organ transplantion, or certain rheumatologic conditions and their respective treatments).

DIAGNOSIS

In addition to a consistent history and physical examination, diagnostic tests for TB have relied on rather old methods including the tuberculin skin test (TST) and microscopic analysis and culture of infected body fluids. A skin test is considered positive if there are 10 millimeters or more of induration at 48 to 72 hours when interpreted by a qualified reader. In close contacts of infected patients, a skin test reaction of 5 millimeters or more of induration is considered positive. A positive test only signifies infection with *M. tuberculosis*. The presence of disease from this organism still has to be further evaluated with a chest X-ray and physician evaluation.

Underlying conditions may suppress the skin test reaction; therefore, if the diagnosis of tuberculosis is strongly suspected, other methods of diagnosis must be pursued. Microscopic demonstration of *M. tuberculosis* in sputum, gastric aspirates, or other body fluids or tissues and isolation in culture are the definitive diagnostic techniques. Occasionally, skin test results are equivocal and must be repeated in 3 months. There is insufficient experience with the QuantiFERON Gold blood test in children to use it at this time for diagnosis, especially in children less than 5 years of age.

TREATMENT

Treatment of TB in children depends on the disease classification (latent infection versus disease) and the anatomic location of disease. Children with latent TB infection, characterized by exposure but a lack of disease, a positive skin test, and a normal chest X-ray, can be treated with a single drug, isoniazid (INH), daily for nine months. Children who do not have a normal immune system (from HIV or other medical conditions) may need a longer course of treatment. Children who have active TB disease are treated with a combination drug regimen which usually consists of three or four drugs: isoniazid (INH), rifampin, pyrazinamide, and sometimes ethambutol. Typically all drugs are taken for the first two months of treatment, followed by a two-drug regimen (INH and rifampin) for an additional four months to complete a total of six months of therapy. These medications are given daily for the first 4 to 8 weeks. Because the mycobacteria are so slow-growing, the medications may be given twice a week for the remainder of the course. Twice a week regimens are particularly advantageous for those families in whom compliance cannot be assured, as it is then feasible for school, childcare, or public health workers actually to administer the medications. However, these intermittent doses can only be administered under a directly observed therapy (DOT) program in which a member of the public health department administers the medications. Consistent implementation of directly observed therapy (DOT) programs has been one of the most important factors responsible for the decrease in new cases and drug-resistant strains in the United States; this strategy has been endorsed by the World Health Organization.

Children with extensive disease (e.g., severe pulmonary involvement, miliary tuberculosis, meningitis, bone infection) or suspected drug resistance, are usually hospitalized for the first several days or weeks of the illness. Once the disease process has been controlled, therapy may be completed as an outpatient. The course of therapy may be extended to 12 to 18 months, depending on the clinical response and the susceptibility of the organisms to the drugs used. Surgical drainage of infection may be required, particularly in cases of bone or joint involvement. A prescribed course of therapy must be completed in order to prevent relapse or disseminated disease. Young infants with asymptomatic tuberculous infection are at great risk of developing meningitis or miliary tuberculosis if incompletely treated.

INFECTIOUS PERIOD

Children with asymptomatic or noncavitary lung disease are almost never infectious. Adolescents and adults with cavitary disease are infectious until all three of the following are met:

effective antituberculous therapy has been initiated, the cough has decreased, and there is a diminishing number of organisms identified on acid-fast microscopy stains of their sputum. Infectivity decreases dramatically after just a few days of appropriate therapy and only rarely persists beyond 1 to 2 weeks. Because of the threat of MDR tuberculosis, high-risk patients are considered infectious until there are no organisms seen on acid-fast stains of their sputum.

INFECTION CONTROL

Parental Advice ► The parents should be informed of the situation and educated concerning the risks to their children. A group meeting should be held and parents provided with a written statement that was prepared in collaboration with the public health department and/or a physician who serves in an advisory role for the center or school. It is important that parents are reassured and educated regarding the disease and the common misconceptions that people have about tuberculosis. When the source adult is a family member who has had minimal or no contact with the other children at the center or school and is not a teacher or childcare worker, it should be emphasized that skin testing is a conservative precaution, and the risk of infection in the children is minimal. New enrollees should not be accepted until the tuberculin status of all adult childcare workers has been determined.

Vaccine ► The BCG vaccines are derived from an attenuated strain of *M. bovis*, a closely related organism to *M. tuberculosis*, and are effective in preventing disseminated forms of disease resulting from *M. tuberculous* infection. These vaccines are used routinely in all newborns only in areas of the world where the rates of disease are high and surveillance and treatment of infected individuals are not possible. In the United States, this vaccine is not routinely used.

Exclusion from Daycare or Preschool Attendance ► Infants and children with tuberculosis may attend the childcare setting as long as they are receiving appropriate therapy according to a carefully formulated plan. The normal level of activities may be resumed once symptoms have disappeared.

Infants and children with draining wounds require a physician's statement that the drainage is no longer infectious. It is critical to keep in mind that children with tuberculosis typically have been recently infected from an adult or adolescent. Therefore, limited exposure of other daycare members to this potentially infectious adult/adolescent is the most important control measure until all contact investigations have been completed and treatments initiated.

Recommendations for Other Children ▶ In the 1960s and 1970s, the incidence of TB was quite high and it was recommended that all children get screened for latent TB infection with a tuberculin skin test. However, now that the incidence has declined, recommendations have shifted to performing targeted TB screening among high-risk children. A child at high risk has more than one of the following: birth outside of the United States, travel outside of the United States, exposure to anyone with TB, close contact with anyone with a positive tuberculin skin test result, close contact with anyone who has been in jail, shelters, uses illegal drugs, or has HIV, consumption of raw milk/unpasteurized cheeses, residence with someone who was born or travelled outside of the United States. A child with more than one risk factor should be screened. If the screening test is positive, the child should be evaluated by a physician. A contact investigation should be conducted to best determine the infectious source.

If a case of active TB is present at the center, the public health department should be notified and will assist in completing the contact investigation. Extent of exposure of the other children to the source adult case will determine the extent of screening:

- If the source adult is a childcare worker or a family member who has had regular close contact with the children, the exposure is high-risk, similar to that of household contacts. All children less than 4 years of age are skin tested, have a chest X-ray performed, and begin INH preventive therapy. Any child with a negative skin test is retested at 12 weeks. If the test remains negative, the initial chest X-ray was negative, and the child is well, INH is discontinued. If either the first or second skin test is positive, INH is continued for at least 9 months. Children 4 years or older do not require INH preventive therapy in the absence of an initial positive skin test, but should be retested after 12 weeks.

- If the source adult is a household contact of the infected child and has had limited or no exposure to the other children in the center, the risk of infection is minimal. All children are skin tested initially. Children with positive skin tests receive a chest X-ray and INH for at least 9 months. Repeated skin testing at 12 weeks for those children who are initially negative is not recommended unless other family members with regular exposure to the childcare center or other childcare center attendees were discovered to have active tuberculosis during the contact investigation.

- Alternative preventive drugs will be considered if the first case is infected with an MDR strain of *M. tuberculosis*.

Recommendations for Personnel ► Childcare workers should be screened with a tuberculin skin test prior to employment. In the home daycare setting, all household members must be included for screening even if some individuals will not be caring for the children directly. Any person with a positive skin test requires a chest X-ray and physician evaluation. If a staff member with active tuberculosis disease is identified, he or she should be reported to the public health department, treated, and excluded from the daycare center or preschool until no longer considered infectious by the supervising physician. A complete contact investigation must be performed. As for the children, the extent of contact with the source adult determines the extent of diagnostic screening that is recommended. If there has been frequent exposure to the source adult, initial skin testing is performed and, if negative, repeated at 12 weeks. Initiation of INH preventive therapy for adults with a negative initial skin test is indicated only for individuals who have impaired immunity while awaiting results of the second skin test. Pregnant women are evaluated as healthy adults and are treated only when definite *M. tuberculosis* disease has been diagnosed. INH prophylaxis for a positive skin test in the absence of disease may be deferred until after delivery unless there has been recent contact with an infectious person. If extent of exposure to the source adult is unclear, a single skin testing is recommended.

67

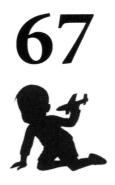

VARICELLA-ZOSTER VIRUS

(Chickenpox, Shingles)

Anne A. Gershon

SIGNS AND SYMPTOMS

Varicella (chickenpox) is the first infection with the varicella-zoster virus (VZV). In the prevaccine era, it usually occurred in children younger than 10 years of age; today it may develop in any age group, including older children and even adults. Symptoms include a rash that begins with raised red lesions that rapidly progress to vesicles, pustules, and crusts. The lesions are most concentrated on the trunk, face, and scalp. They are intensely itchy. The illness is often accompanied by fever and lasts for about 5 days. Varicella infection without any signs or symptoms is believed to occur in about 5 percent of cases. The major complication in otherwise healthy persons is bacterial superinfection (especially with group A streptococci) of the skin. The disease is usually benign in children, unless they are immunocompromised. In severe cases, the lesions may number in the thousands and become hemorrhagic. Varicella pneumonia is a serious complication in such patients. Generally, the extent of the skin rash is a good indication of the mildness or severity of a case of varicella; the more severe the illness, the greater the number of skin lesions. The average child with chickenpox develops 250 to 500 vesicles over about 5 days.

Zoster (shingles) is a secondary infection with VZV. It only occurs in persons who have experienced a previous episode of either clinical or subclinical varicella, or, rarely, in individuals who have been vaccinated. The virus becomes latent in the sensory nerves during chickenpox and may remain latent for months to years. Latency probably occurs much more commonly after natural infection than vaccination. In shingles, the virus infects a dermatomal (an area of skin enervated by one nerve) area of skin, resulting in a unilateral localized vesicular rash that may be painful. Zoster is most common in immuno-compromised patients and the elderly, although children may manifest it. Children seem to be at increased risk for zoster if, while they were in utero, their mothers had varicella or they had varicella before 1 year of age. Zoster in childhood is usually a mild self-limited illness unless the child is immuno-compromised.

CAUSE

VZV is a herpes virus closely related to other agents such as herpes simplex virus (HSV), cytomegalovirus, and Epstein–Barr virus (EBV). There is only one serotype. There is no cross-protection among these agents. All of the herpes viruses become latent after primary infection and may later reactivate. VZV and HSV become latent in sensory nerves.

SPREAD AND CONTROL

Source of the Organism ▸ The major source of VZV is the skin lesions of both varicella and zoster, which, when moist, are full of infectious viral particles. Presumably, the virus becomes aerosolized when patients scratch the skin lesions. Although it is almost impossible to culture VZV from respiratory secretions, the respiratory tract is also possibly a source of infectious virus, and children are believed to be at least somewhat contagious to others 1 to 2 days before developing the chickenpox rash. Varicella is extremely contagious, but zoster is less so.

High-Risk Populations ► Individuals who have not previously been vaccinated or infected with natural VZV and who therefore have no immunity to VZV are at risk to develop chickenpox following exposure to someone with either varicella or zoster. Second attacks of varicella are unusual, and if they occur, they are likely to be mild. Mild cases of varicella are thought to occur in 10 to 15 percent of vaccinated children following close exposure to individuals infected with the natural virus. Subclinical reinfection of persons who have had varicella is common following subsequent exposure.

Patients with immune deficiencies are at additional risk to develop severe varicella if they have not had the infection previously. Newborn infants whose mothers have the onset of varicella between 5 days before and 2 days after delivery are also at high risk to develop severe varicella. They should be given immunoglobulin and/or antiviral therapy (see Treatment recommendations).

Mode of Spread ► The virus is spread by the airborne route. Chickenpox is not spread by contaminated environmental articles but requires person-to-person contact. In family settings, the attack rate among susceptibles is 80 to 90 percent. Transmission after less intimate exposures (such as in school) is less predictable. The disease is not transmissible until 1 to 2 days prior to development of rash, and it remains transmissible until the skin lesions have crusted. Vaccinated children who nevertheless develop varicella are contagious to others. There is a general direct relationship between the number of skin lesions present and the degree of contagion.

Incubation Period ► Ten to 21 days.

DIAGNOSIS

The diagnosis of both chickenpox and shingles can usually be made on clinical grounds based on the history of contact and the nature and distribution of the rash. When the rash is not characteristic of varicella, a scraping of a skin lesion can be obtained for staining. Increasingly, polymerase chain reaction (PCR) is becoming more available for laboratory diagnosis of

VZV infections; this assay is highly sensitive and practical. It may be used not only to identify VZV infection but also to determine whether the infection is due to the natural virus or the vaccine (Oka) strain. Skin lesions may also be cultured for the presence of virus, but today this test is rarely used, due to both lack of sensitivity and the expense. Antibody titers for VZV antibodies may also be obtained, but the diagnosis cannot be made for at least 7 to 10 days after the onset of illness by this method. The diagnosis of zoster can be made on similar grounds. There is no need to elicit a history of contact with someone with VZV, however, as zoster is the result of reactivation of latent infection in the patient.

TREATMENT

The oral administration of acyclovir (ACV) to children and adolescents within 24 hours after onset of the rash of chickenpox shortens the course of the illness in children by about a day. The American Academy of Pediatrics has published recommendations for use of ACV in children with chickenpox. One approach is to administer it to children over age 12 years and to secondary household cases that are predictably more severe than the primary case in a family. It is not recommended that ACV be given to try to prevent varicella from developing if an exposure has been recognized. Antiviral therapy is usually unnecessary for vaccinated children who develop breakthrough varicella as this is typically a mild disease.

Immunocompromised children with no history of varicella should be given VZV antibodies, VariZIG, which has supplanted varicella-zoster immune globulin (VZIG) within 3 (maximum, 5) days of a close exposure to someone with either chickenpox or shingles. Infants born to women with the onset of varicella 5 days before delivery to 2 days after delivery should also receive VariZIG.

Children who develop severe varicella should be treated with intravenous ACV. Immunocompromised children who develop varicella and have not received either VZIG or varicella vaccine (see below) should also be treated with intravenous ACV as early in the illness as possible, even if the disease is mild and there are few skin lesions, mainly to prevent the development of varicella pneumonia.

Usually, shingles in children does not require therapy, as it is a self-limited illness. Exceptions include zoster of the eye and zoster in an immunocompromised child. Each case requires individualization.

INFECTIOUS PERIOD

Patients with varicella and zoster are infectious to others until all the skin lesions have crusted; usually this occurs within 5 to 7 days, but it may be longer in immunosuppressed patients.

INFECTION CONTROL

Parental Advice ▶ Parents should be notified of the occurrence of varicella in an attendee or staff member in case there is a varicella-susceptible pregnant woman or immunocompromised person in the family.

Vaccine ▶ A live attenuated varicella vaccine (Oka strain) was licensed by the U.S. Food and Drug Administration for use in all children over the age of 12 months and for adults who are susceptible to chickenpox in March 1995. It is recommended by both the American Academy of Pediatrics and the Centers for Disease Control and Prevention that the vaccine be given routinely to all who are susceptible. The vaccine is extremely safe and effective for prevention of most cases of varicella. One dose is recommended for children from 1 to 12 years of age, a second dose should be at least 4 weeks after the first dose was given; intervals can vary from weeks to 4 to 6 years of age. As the vaccine cannot be given to pregnant women, and because it is recommended that women not become pregnant until at least 3 months after a dose of varicella vaccine, it is particularly important to determine if women of childbearing age with no history of varicella have detectable immunity. Administration of vaccine inadvertently to persons who are immune to varicella is not harmful.

Exclusion from Daycare or Preschool Attendance ▶ Children with acute natural (wild-type) chickenpox should not attend daycare or preschool until all the lesions have crusted. This usually leads to exclusion for about 5 to 7 days. The rare child with shingles can attend daycare or preschool if the skin lesions are on the trunk and can be fully covered with a sterile dressing and clothing.

Children who were immunized may develop a rash during the 6 weeks following immunization. Only 5 percent of vaccinated children develop a rash, and most of these rashes consist of only a few lesions that resemble insect bites. Although these children with rash may potentially transmit vaccine-type VZV to others, transmission of vaccine-type virus is highly unlikely. It should be remembered, however, that until there is universal use of varicella vaccine with resultant little circulation of wild-type VZV, some children with apparent vaccine-associated rashes may actually be in the early stages of natural varicella that was in the incubation period when they were immunized. Thus, vaccinated children who develop vesicles suggestive of varicella should not attend daycare until the vesicles are dried or a diagnosis other than varicella is made, particularly in the first 2 weeks after vaccination. Transmission of vaccine-type virus is less dangerous than transmission of wild-type VZV. It appears that the vaccine-type virus is much less able to result in transmission and, when transmission occurs, the resultant illness is a very modified form of varicella due to the attenuated nature of the vaccine-type virus. In general, these recommendations also apply to adults who have recently been immunized. It is strongly recommended that daycare and preschool facilities prospectively develop their own policies for potential management of vaccinated children and adults; these will need to be modified periodically as the vaccine is more widely implemented.

Routine use of varicella vaccine should prevent most disease in child daycare settings. However, outbreaks due to the natural virus in vaccinated children in daycare have been observed. Presumably, these infrequent occurrences are in children who did not respond to the vaccine or, rarely, are possibly due to waning immunity. Although it is rare, zoster has been reported in children who have been vaccinated. This is due to vaccine virus in one third and wild-type natural VZV in two thirds of these children. Vaccinees with zoster can transmit varicella to susceptible children and adults.

Administration of vaccine to susceptibles who have already been exposed is now acceptable ("post-exposure prophylaxis"). Varicella vaccine has been useful in terminating outbreaks of the infection, including those occurring in daycare settings. It is not necessary to administer additional vaccine to children who have already had 2 doses should an exposure occur.

Recommendations for Other Children ► Passive immunization with immunoglobulin is recommended only for immunocompromised children at high risk to develop severe varicella.

Recommendations for Personnel ► Adults who have never had varicella should be immunized before being exposed to VZV. Adults should be given 2 doses of vaccine 4 to 8 weeks apart. This will result in immunity to varicella in about 90 percent of adults. Those who do not develop detectable antibodies after 2 doses may be given a third dose and be retested for development of antibodies, but it should be recalled that most available serologic tests lack sensitivity for this purpose. Adults who fail to develop antibodies (seroconvert) after 3 doses of vaccine are unlikely to respond to a fourth dose. Most adults who seroconvert after two doses can be expected to be protected against varicella; about 10 percent may develop modified varicella with an average of 50 skin lesions and rapid recovery. Adult vaccinees who remain seropositive are highly unlikely to develop breakthrough varicella following exposure to the wild-type virus. Varicella-susceptible pregnant women who develop wild-type chickenpox in the first or second trimester of pregnancy have a 2 percent risk of delivering a child with the characteristic constellation of birth defects (skin, nervous system, and eyes) of the congenital varicella syndrome. This syndrome has not been observed to be caused by the vaccine-type virus.

68

YERSINIA

Barbara A. Jantausch
William J. Rodriguez

SIGNS AND SYMPTOMS

Yersinia pestis is responsible for human plague. *Yersinia entero-colitica* and *Yersinia pseudotuberculosis* cause gastrointestinal illness that is collectively called yersiniosis. *Y. enterocolitica* primarily causes diarrhea, nausea, and fever and also can cause mesenteric adenitis. It is the cause of large epidemics of gastroenteritis. Children with *Y. enterocolitica* infections may have fever to 104°F with bloody diarrhea, nausea, vomiting, and colicky abdominal pain. Stools may be watery but are more often mucousy. Illness may last from a few days to 1 month, but it usually is present for less than 10 days. Infection may be asymptomatic. *Y. pseudotuberculosis* causes abdominal pain and mesenteric adenitis. *Y. enterocolitica* and *Y. pseudotuber-culosis* can be responsible for a pseudoappendicitis syndrome, prompting appendectomy that in most cases yields a normal appendix and suppurative mesenteric lymph nodes.

Extraintestinal manifestations of yersinia infections may include arthritis, erythema nodosum, Reiter's syndrome, low platelet count, bloodstream infection, and meningitis. Asymptomatic infections occur rarely.

CAUSE

Yersinia is a gastrointestinal gram-negative bacillus. There are three species: *Y. pestis, Y. enterocolitica,* and *Y. pseudotuberculosis.*

SPREAD AND CONTROL

Source of the Organism ► Primary reservoirs for yersinia are contaminated food and water and animal carriers, specifically, dogs, cats (especially those who have stayed in animal shelters), pigs, cows, goats, horses, rabbits, squirrels, rodents, domestic fowl, and fish. A recognized cause of yersiniosis in young infants is contact with an adult who has handled pork intestines (chitterlings). *Y. enterocolitica* is more common in winter than summer.

High-Risk Populations ► Children with hemolytic conditions (e.g., sickle cell anemia), that lead to increased storage of iron may be at high risk, as are those on immunosuppressive therapy.

Mode of Spread ► Food or water contaminated by feces or urine from animals is probably the main mode of spread; others include the fecal–oral route and person-to-person transmission. The organism is able to survive in refrigerated milk.

Incubation Period ► The incubation period is 2 to 11 days, with an average of 5 days, but may extend up to 3 weeks.

DIAGNOSIS

Y. enterocolitica may be isolated from stool cultures. *Y. pseudotuberculosis* is rarely recovered from stool cultures; in cases of mesenteric adenitis it has been grown from infected lymph nodes. In disseminated infection, Yersinia can be readily recovered from blood or other body fluids using standard culture techniques. A four-fold rise in antibody titer specific against the offending serotype can be diagnostic.

TREATMENT

Despite the fact that antibiotic therapy has not proved to be definitively effective in *Y. enterocolitica* enterocolitis, we would recommend the use of effective oral antimicrobial agents in symptomatic patients. *Y. enterocolitica* is usually sensitive to aminoglycosides, third-generation cephalosporins, chloramphenicol, fluoroquinolones, and trimethoprim-sulfamethoxazole. For those older than 9 years of age, tetracyclines can be used if the organism is susceptible. Treatment of enteric disease without invasion should be with absorbable antimicrobials for 5 to 7 days. Patients with bloodstream or disseminated infection may require intravenous or intramuscular antibiotic therapy for a longer period of time.

INFECTIOUS PERIOD

Y. enterocolitica has been recovered from the stool 4 to 79 days (average, 27 days) after symptoms have resolved and for as long as 6 weeks after antimicrobial therapy.

INFECTION CONTROL

Parental Advice ► Parents should observe their child for symptoms of enteritis. Symptomatic children should be removed from daycare, seen by their pediatrician, and have their stools cultured. The physician should be informed of the presence of yersinia at the daycare center or preschool.

Vaccine ► None available.

Exclusion from Daycare or Preschool Attendance ► Although the period of communicability is unknown and patients may shed the organism even after antibiotic therapy is completed, it seems reasonable to keep the child out of the center only while symptomatic.

Recommendations for Other Children ► Children should avoid contact with feces. Other children in the setting who become symptomatic with diarrhea should be removed from the setting and have their stools cultured for yersinia.

Recommendations for Personnel ▶ Personnel who become symptomatic should remain at home and have their stools cultured for yersinia. All personnel should practice good hand-washing. Diapers should be disposed of properly, and separate diaper and food preparation areas provided. Toys that the infected child played with should be disinfected. New children should not be enrolled during an outbreak.

AFTERWORD

The aim of this book is to provide you, the parents, with a ready reference guide to the following questions:

- What are the infections in daycare and preschool?
- How are these infections spread?
- What are the best practices that the daycare or preschool can and should use to minimize infectious illnesses and the spread of germs?
- What should be done when infections do occur in the center or preschool?
- What should I expect and what should be done when my child has an infection?

"Dr. Google" is not a reliable source of medical information for your child. At all times, your child's doctor is the one who knows you and your child, and is the best, most consistent, and most dedicated resource to prevent and diagnose illness, and to counsel you on your child's healthcare needs.

Leigh B. Grossman, MD

INDEX

Page numbers followed by QR *indicate Quick References.*

Body Lice, 252–256. *See also* Lice
  (pediculosis)
Boils, Staphylococcal, 309–313
Bordetella pertussis. *See* Pertussis
  (Whooping Cough)
Brain injuries. *See* Children with
  disabilities
Breastfeeding
  antibody transmission through,
    285
  HIV transmission through, 203
Breathing, rapid or altered, 9QR, 74,
    88, 135, 258, 270
Bronchiolitis
  in Adenovirus infection, 111
  in pneumonia, 233
  in Respiratory Syncytial Virus
    infection, 270
Bronchitis, 57QR
  in Adenovirus infection, 111
  in Pneumococcal infection, 57
  treatment, 38–39
Bronchopulmonary Dysplasia
  (BPD), 87–89
Burkholderia cepacia, 88

Calcivirus, transmission, 13QR
Campylobacter, 13QR, 52QR,
    127–130
  cause, 128
  diagnosis, 129
  exclusion recommendations, 52,
    130
  incubation period, 52, 129
  infection control, 128–130
  infectious period, 130
  parental care recommendations,
    130
  personnel care recommenda-
    tions, 130
  signs and symptoms, 127–128
  transmission of, 13, 52, 128–129

treatment, 129–130
Cancer
  common infections, 78, 79
  exclusion recommendations, 85
  infection control, 79–81
  infectious risks, 77–78
  parental care recommendations,
    84–85
  in personnel, 22
  personnel care recommenda-
    tions, 84–85
  risks to healthy children, 81–84
  risk to other children, 81
Candida, 131–134
  diagnosis, 133
  exclusion recommendations, 134
  in HIV infection, 201
  in immunodeficient children, 82
  infection control, 132–134
  infectious period, 133
  oral, 131
  parental care recommendations,
    133
  personnel care recommenda-
    tions, 134
  risk to other children, 134
  signs and symptoms, 131–132
  transmission, 132–133
  treatment, 133
Cardiac disease. *See* Congenital
  Heart Disease
Catheters, infection control for,
    80–81
Cellulitis
  in children with disabilities, 95
  in *H. influenzae* infection,
    176–183
  in Staphylococcal infection,
    309–313
  in Streptococcal infection,
    314–318

Cerebral palsy. *See* Children with
  disabilities
Chancre, in Syphilis, 320, 321
Chemotherapy, infection risk and,
  267
Chickenpox (Varicella), 13QR,
  30QR, 52QR, 59, 346–352
  cause, 347
  diagnosis, 348–349
  exclusion recommendations, 52,
    59–60, 85, 350–352
  in immunosuppressed children,
    79–80, 82–83
  incubation period, 52, 59, 348
  infection control, 347–348,
    350–352
  infectious period, 350
  parental care recommendations,
    350
  personnel care recommenda-
    tions, 352
  risk to other children, 352
  signs and symptoms, 59–60,
    346–347
  transmission, 13, 52, 347–348
  treatment, 349–350
  vaccination, 350–352
    of immunosuppressed chil-
      dren, 91
    of personnel, 23, 25
    recommended schedule, 30
Child Care Center. *See* Daycare
  Center
Children with disabilities, 92–98
  common infections, 94–95
  exclusion recommendations, 97
  infection control, 95–98
  infectious risks, 93
  parental care recommendations,
    98
  personnel care recommenda-
    tions, 97–98
  risk of infections, 93

risks to healthy children, 96–97
  well childcare, 93
Chlamydia, 135–138
  diagnosis, 137
  exclusion recommendations, 138
  incubation period, 137
  infection control, 136–138
  infectious period, 138
  parental care recommendations,
    138
  personnel care recommenda-
    tions, 138
  risk to other children, 138
  signs and symptoms, 135
  transmission, 136–137
  treatment, 137–138
Cirrhosis
  in Hepatitis B infection, 188, 190
  in Hepatitis C infection, 193
Cleaning procedures, 26–27, 45QR
  bedding, 27
  blood-contaminated surfaces,
    208
  carpets, 27
  contaminated surfaces, 26–27
  in epidemics, 45
  in infant care, 73
  toys and play equipment, 27
Cleft palate, ear infections, 94
Cognitive impairment, 25, 92, 95,
    96, 189, 192. *See also* Chil-
    dren with disabilities
Cold, Common, 13QR, 57QR,
    276–278
  in Adenovirus infection, 111
  causative agents, 37
  cause, 139, 277
  in Coronavirus infection,
    139–140
  diagnosis, 37, 140, 277
  ear infection with, 37
  exclusion recommendations, 140,
    278

for Campylobacter infection, 52,
130
for cancer, 85
for Candida infection, 134
for Chickenpox (Varicella) infection, 52, 59–60, 85, 350–352
for children with disabilities, 97
for Chlamydia infection, 138
for common cold, 278
for conjunctivitis (Pink Eye), 52,
60
for Coronavirus infection, 140
for Cryptosporidium infection,
146
for Cytomegalovirus infection,
53, 60, 150
for diarrhea, 60
for Diphtheria infection, 154
for *E. coli* infection, 53, 166
for Enterovirus infection, 162
for Erythema infectiosum (Fifth
Disease), 53, 60, 250–251
for Giardia infection, 53, 61, 170
for Gingivostomatitis (Herpes
Simplex virus), 54, 61
for Gonorrhea infection, 174
for Hand, Foot, and Mouth
Syndrome (Coxsackievirus
A16), 54, 61, 143
for Hepatitis A virus (HAV)
infection, 54, 61, 187
for Hepatitis B virus (HBV) infection, 54, 61, 191–192
for Hepatitis C virus (HCV)
infection, 195
for Herpes Simplex virus infection, 96, 198
for *H. influenzae* infection, 180
for HIV infection and AIDS
infection, 85, 207–208
for Hookworm infection, 239
for immunocompromised and
immunodeficient children,
85

for impetigo, 55, 62
for infants, 73–74
for Influenza infection, 54–55,
62, 217–218
for Lice infestation, 55, 62, 256
for lung disease, 88
for Measles (Rubeola) infection,
55, 62, 85, 296
for Meningococcal infection, 56,
62, 222
for *Molluscum contagiosum* infection, 226
for Mononucleosis, 55, 62, 213
for Mycoplasma infection, 235
for Mumps infection, 56, 63, 230
for Pertussis (Whooping Cough)
infection, 58, 64, 263–264
for Papillomavirus infection, 243
for Parainfluenza virus infection,
246
for Pinworm infection, 56, 159
for Pneumococcal infection, 57,
269
for respiratory infection, 57, 63
for Respiratory Syncytial Virus
infection, 274
for Roseola infection, 57, 63, 282
for Rotavirus infection, 57, 63,
286
for Roundworm (*A. lumbricoides*) infection, 126
for Rubella (German Measles)
infection, 53, 60, 290
for Salmonella infection, 57, 301
for Scabies infestation, 58, 63, 304
for Scarlet Fever, 58, 63–64
for Shigella infection, 58, 308
for skin disease, chronic, 100
for sore throat, 56, 63–64
for Staphylococcal infection, 55,
312
for Streptococcal infection,
317–318

77307036R00231

Made in the USA
Lexington, KY
26 December 2017